A Chaplain's Expertise

(A New Paradigm)

by

Rev. John Skanse,

MDiv., COL ILANG (Retired), BCC

A CHAPLAIN'S EXPERTISE (A NEW PARADIGM)

1405 SW 6th Avenue • Ocala, Florida 34471 • Phone 800-814-1132 • Fax 352-622-1875
Website: www.atlantic-pub.com • Email: sales@atlantic-pub.com
SAN Number: 268-1250

Library of Congress Cataloging-in-Publication Data

Names: Skanse, John, 1950- author.
Title: A chaplain's expertise : a new paradigm / by Rev. John Skanse, MDiv., COL ILANG (Retired), BCC.
Description: Ocala : Atlantic Publishing Group, Inc., 2018. | Includes bibliographical references and index.
Identifiers: LCCN 2017055431 (print) | LCCN 2017057850 (ebook) | ISBN 9781620235201 (ebook) | ISBN 9781620235195 (pbk. : alk. paper) | ISBN 1620235196 (alk. paper)
Subjects: LCSH: Chaplains. | Pastoral medicine. | Chaplains, Hospital. | Church work with the sick.
Classification: LCC BV4375 (ebook) | LCC BV4375 .S53 2018 (print) | DDC 259/.4—dc23
LC record available at https://lccn.loc.gov/2017055431

Printed in the United States

PROJECT MANAGER: Danielle Lieneman
INTERIOR LAYOUT: Nicole Sturk

Reduce. Reuse. RECYCLE.

A decade ago, Atlantic Publishing signed the Green Press Initiative. These guidelines promote environmentally friendly practices, such as using recycled stock and vegetable-based inks, avoiding waste, choosing energy-efficient resources, and promoting a no-pulping policy. We now use 100-percent recycled stock on all our books. The results: in one year, switching to post-consumer recycled stock saved 24 mature trees, 5,000 gallons of water, the equivalent of the total energy used for one home in a year, and the equivalent of the greenhouse gases from one car driven for a year.

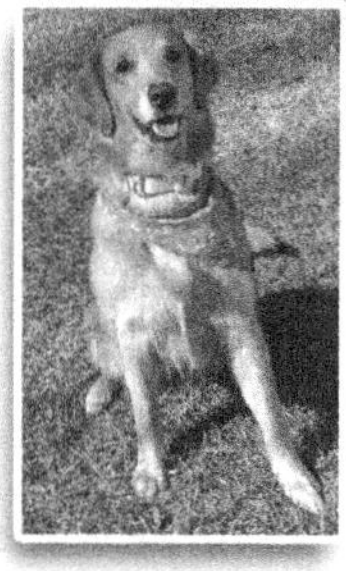
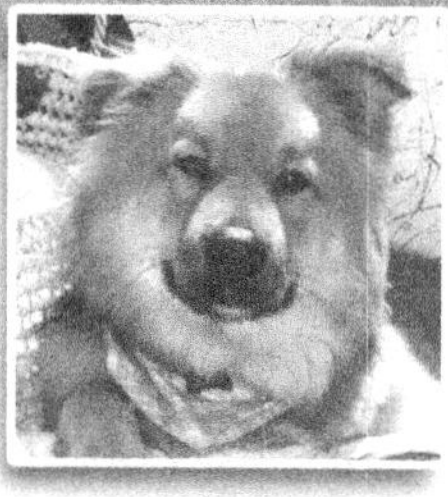
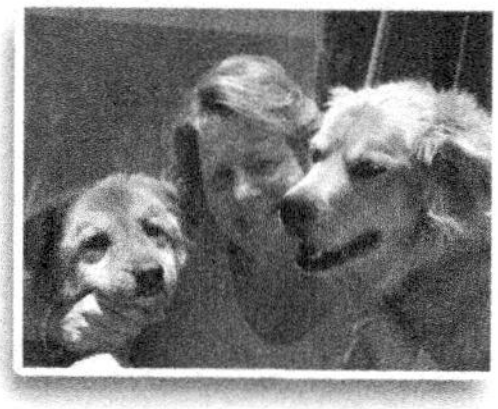

Over the years, we have adopted a number of dogs from rescues and shelters. First there was Bear and after he passed, Ginger and Scout. Now, we have Kira, another rescue. They have brought immense joy and love not just into our lives, but into the lives of all who met them.

We want you to know a portion of the profits of this book will be donated in Bear, Ginger and Scout's memory to local animal shelters, parks, conservation organizations, and other individuals and nonprofit organizations in need of assistance.

– Douglas & Sherri Brown,

President & Vice-President of Atlantic Publishing

A Chaplain's Expertise

(A New Paradigm)

by

Rev. John Skanse,

MDiv., COL ILANG (Retired), BCC

January 2018

Table of Contents

Preface

Much has been written about chaplaincy, each work helping to express and develop a piece of understanding about how and why a chaplain's function is of such importance in the care of people in medical and other settings.

Themes like "The Living Human Document"[1], "The Courageous Shepherd"[2], "The Wounded Healer"[3], "The Circus Clown"[4], "The Intimate Stranger"[5], "The Diagnostician"[6], "The Agent of Hope"[7], and others have been explored and presented as ways of developing and understanding chaplaincy.

---

1. Boisen, A. T. (2005). The Living Human Document. In Robert C. Dykstra (Ed.), *Images of Pastoral Care, Classic Readings* (pp.22-29). St. Louis, Missouri: Chalice Press.
2. Campbell, A. V. (2005). The Courageous Shepherd. In Robert C. Dykstra (Ed.), *Images of Pastoral Care, Classic Readings* (pp.54-61). St. Louis, Missouri: Chalice Press.
3. Nouwen, H. J. M. (2005). The Wounded Healer. In Robert C. Dykstra (Ed.), *Images of Pastoral Care, Classic Readings* (pp.76-84). St. Louis, Missouri: Chalice Press.
4. Faber, H (2005). The Circus Clown. In Robert C. Dykstra (Ed.), *Images of Pastoral Care, Classic Readings* (pp.85-93). St. Louis, Missouri: Chalice Press.
5. Dykstra, R. C. (2005). The Intimate Stranger. In Robert C. Dykstra (Ed.), *Images of Pastoral Care, Classic Readings* (pp.123-136). St. Louis, Missouri: Chalice Press.
6. Pruyser, P. W. (2005). The Diagnostician. In Robert C. Dykstra (Ed.), *Images of Pastoral Care, Classic Readings* (pp.161-170). St. Louis, Missouri: Chalice Press.
7. Capps, D. (2005). The Agent of Hope. In Robert C. Dykstra (Ed.), *Images of Pastoral Care, Classic Readings* (pp.188-199). St. Louis, Missouri: Chalice Press.

While these, and many other concepts, have been very helpful in exploring the depths of chaplains' duties and their value in society, they lack a common language that can be easily understood across a wide range of society. We, as chaplains, have developed a language of our own that creates little interest and is easily cast off or ignored by the very ones we are trying to help.

As Rev. George Handzo said in his book, *Professional Spiritual and Pastoral Care*, "One of the major barriers to advancing the practice of spiritual care is a lack of definitional clarity among practitioners themselves."[8] The real problem of defining the value of chaplaincy is that we fail to define ourselves in a language easily understood by common society. We speak our own chaplain language, religious language, medical, and business languages that contain their own meanings and cultural variations. Even when using the same words as everyone else, those words can have very different meanings when spoken by people from different groups.

First, and foremost, our focus lies with the patient, and their family and friends. Next, we care for the medical staff who have their own set of concerns. Then, we hope to connect and strengthen the patient's relationship with their clergy and additional resources while in and after hospitalization. Finally, we work under administrators who allow us to be involved with patients and who also pay our salaries, and therefore need to understand fully our value to the medical effort.

In today's volatile economy, as chaplaincy positions are being lost, made part-time or volunteer only, the need to be able to explain the importance of chaplaincy involvement in words most easily understood by all those impacted has become even more pressing; especially in the "patient-centered" milieu of today's medical reality.[9] "Patient satisfaction" has become the bottom line for determining whether care is being delivered properly.

8. Roberts, S. B. (2012). Professional Spiritual & Pastoral Care (p. 24). Skylight Paths Publishing, Woodstock, Vermont: Skylight Paths Publishing.
9. Epstien, R. M. & Street, R. L. Jr. (2011). The Values and Value of Patient-Centered Care. Annals of Family Medicine, 9/2, 100-103.

Most patient surveys concerning care focus on how well the patient and their family feel they have been cared for. Today, patients control their own care more than ever.

This need for members of the chaplaincy to speak more clearly to members of medicine has been partially recognized, in recent years, as chaplaincy associations have taken up the call to focus on researching the "value added" by chaplaincy since research language is a key language of medicine and science when addressing "best practices."[10] This focus has even ultimately lead to the development of an association known as the "The Spiritual Care Association"that is focused on researching the value that chaplaincy brings to the care of patients and their families[11].

In my inner-city, multi-ethnic, multi-cultural, level-one trauma center setting, introductions are made and followed by a blank stare after I've asked, "Do you know what a chaplain is?" More than half of the time I have been met with a resounding, "No", or a "Yes", when they think I am there to just pray with them.

When it comes to medical staff in this same teaching hospital, the idea of what a chaplain does is often limited to the performance of religious services, if requested, or when a patient is dying.

The same is true for our many religious volunteers, both lay and clergy, when they first become involved in our religious volunteer program. The community clergy do not often realize how much we wish to partner with them and support and add to their efforts in caring for their congregants.

I myself have struggled with the question of what the chaplain's value is and what purpose a chaplain has in a medical setting. I pastored for almost 30 years, served as an Air Force chaplain for 20 years, volunteered as a police

10. Hall, E. J., Hughes, B. P. & Handzo, G. H. (2016, October), Retrieved from https://www.healthcarechaplaincy.org/docs/about/spirituality.pdf
11. About Spiritual Care Association (2017), Retrieved from https://www.spiritualcareassociation.org

chaplain, and taught as an adjunct professor on the psychological aspects of disaster for a few years. Through my variety of experiences, I discovered that in medical settings there are distinct differences, along with similarities, that create the emphatic need for chaplains when caring for people facing the uncertainties of medical care.

The role of a chaplain in medical settings is uniquely different from that of a pastor or chaplain in a congregational, military, or prison setting, most of which are parish oriented. These are settings in which one tries to build and support a group of people around a group of religious doctrines.

The differences of medically oriented spiritual care have been expressed in many ways. These concepts have helped chaplains develop their own ways of functioning but have done little to express to other groups a chaplain's importance.

The language of chaplaincy must find the ability to speak to:

1. The patient, in words common to both of them as to why and for what purposes the chaplain is involved,
2. The medical staff, defining what we do so that the staff can remember, and is more ready and willing to call for a chaplain when needed,
3. The pastor going to a sick congregant and meeting a chaplain there,
4. Hospital administrators, who think in bottom line and administrative terms,
5. And the general public, at large, in the same language that can be understood easily by the everyday man and woman.

We must find common words that speak poignantly to not just the medical teams who focus on research and best practices, but also, administrators who speak best in management terms, to patients and their families who are focused on "What are we going to do now?", to visiting clergy who often do not understand how a chaplain is going to help them care for their congregant, and to care-givers who have a very limited understanding of what a chaplain does.

We speak often of the many "tools", that we discover and carry with us on our "tool belt" as chaplains, and that we can pick from to use to help others. Much time and many pages have been spent defining these tools, but what about the tool belt? Are there any common language concepts upon which we can hang all of the other concepts about chaplaincy and make it easier to remember what is on that "tool belt"? The purpose of this book is to share simple, common concepts that help tie together all that chaplaincy is and does for the care of people, in language that is readily acceptable and understood across a wide variety of social groups. This provides a more effective argument for the needed value added when a chaplain is involved in any situation, and a simple framework upon which to hang all the tools we discover and develop for ourselves. This also provides a focused, functional guide that can help a chaplain be able to walk into any situation and provide care that effectively allows for any needed change in a patient or their families' thinking, for better choices, without stepping on the patient's autonomy. The following is a "fleshing-out" of my initial thoughts first published in the chaplain e-magazine, "Plainviews" in 2010.[12]

A snapshot of chaplaincy

"She was deaf. She was blind. She had just fallen and was probably going to be bedridden from now on. Her husband of 67 years was sitting outside her room on a chair like a guard guarding a treasure. She was in our ED.

What could be done? How could her life be touched and her spirits lifted?

12. Skanse, J. E. (2010). Finding a Reason To Be. Plainviews, 7/18. http://www.plainviews.org

Her husband had said she was repeating over and over again that she "wanted to die." He was struggling with how to express his love to her. At home she could hear a little bit when she had on her one hearing aid, but that was at home. There he had told her of his love for her and how he liked to take care of her because of that love, but she felt now like nothing but a burden to him. So she wanted to die. And therefore he was doing the only thing he could think of: guarding her.

What could a chaplain do . . . what could anyone do? Words could not be heard, a smile could not be seen, but what of the power of touch? That which was lost to a husband sitting outside his wife's room, guarding her.

And so I walked in, pulling the curtain open a little more so that he might see what I was doing and maybe catch on. Touch was the only way I might communicate my care for her . . . them.

I took her hand, determined somehow to touch her spirit. 10 minutes passed and she began to cry and say how she could not see, or hear without her hearing aid that was at home and how she had fallen. I squeezed her hand and she squeezed back with a surprising strength. She let her tears dry and we sat holding hands for another 10 minutes. Two people connected only by touch. She, not knowing who was holding her, and I, not knowing fully what was going on inside.

Then a smile came to her face . . . she seemed to sit up a little bit and said, clearer than anything before, "I'm holding the hand of God." Her spirit had been touched, lifted up and she knew this hand was not there to touch her medically or like a family member, but spiritually.

I hope that in seeing and hearing this, her husband caught on to the power of touch.

Chaplains are present to "be" with people, touching their lives, in the midst of stress and crisis with a hand that speaks of there being more to

> *life than just those biological processes that so easily can get messed up with illness and lost in death. A touch that reminds another of God.*"[13] *

The relationship between chaplain and patient is one that helps people face their uncertainties, discovering the resources that they already have, but may have forgotten in the crisis of the moment. We hope to help them find comfort that uplifts and carries them forward with hope in life's moments of uncertainty or despair.

---

13. Skanse, J. E. (2009). The power of touch. *Plainviews*, 6/18. http://www.plainviews.org

*Direct quote edited for grammar and punctuation.

[illegible]

[illegible]

[illegible] of the moment. [illegible]

[illegible]

Chapter 1

Chaplaincy in Context

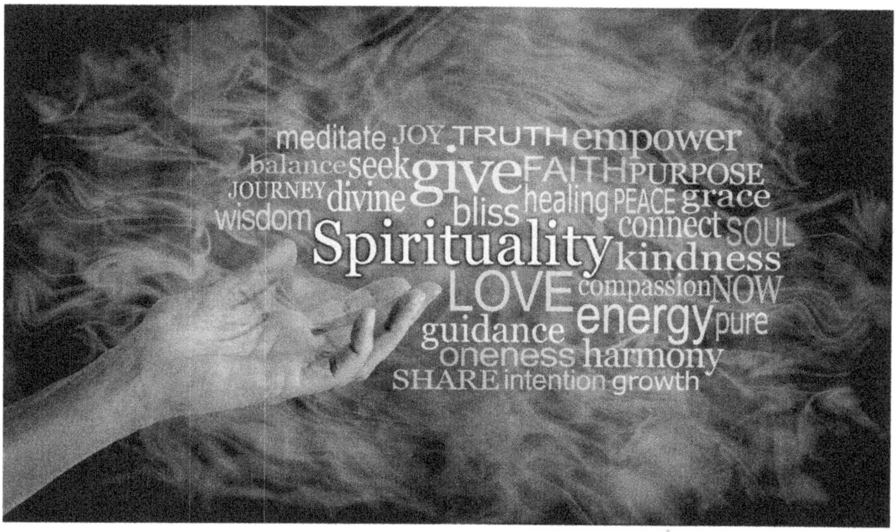

To begin any discussion on chaplaincy we must first put it in the larger context of care.

Chaplaincy focuses on what is often called "spiritual care." This is different than what doctors do for physical care and from psychiatrists and psychologists, who focus on mental and emotional needs. Though different, all of these are closely intermingled. What doctors, psychiatrists, and chaplains do affects how people think and feel, and affects how well a person recovers from the trauma of injury, illness, and imminent death.

Chaplaincy can be viewed from within the psychological spectrum of patient care with a unique focus.

According to the Institute of Transpersonal Psychology:

> *Traditional psychology is interested in a continuum of human experience and behavior ranging from severe dysfunction, mental and emotional illness at one end, to what is generally considered 'normal', healthy behavior at the other end and various degrees of normal and maladjustment in between."*[14]

Figure #1

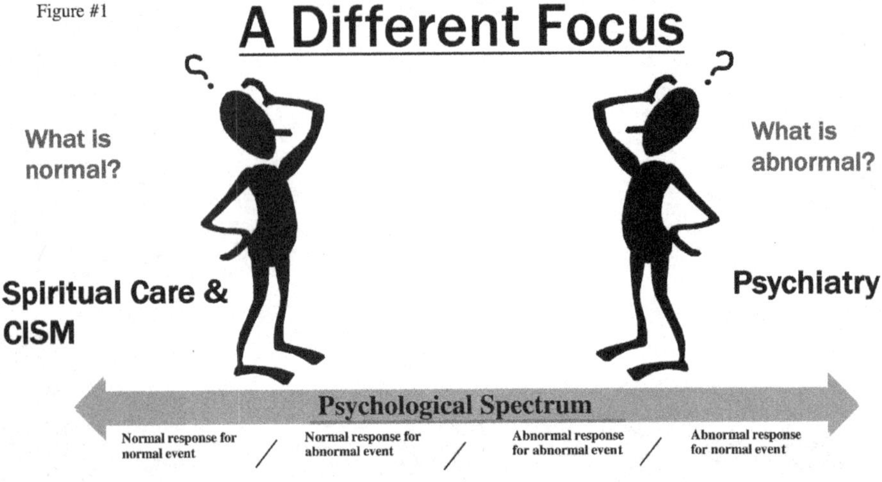

Therefore, one could say that the psychological spectrum runs from "What is normal" to "What is abnormal" (see Figure #1 above). It begins with a person having what they consider a "normal day" in which one has normal responses to normal events, like waking up, going to work, eating lunch, and so on. We might be calmer or more excited about certain happenings during the day but always within a normal range.

14. Tartakovsky, M. (2011, November 03). 6 facts about Transpersonal Psychology [Blog post]. Retrieved from: https://psychcentral.com/blog/archives/2011/11/03/6-facts-about-transpersonal-psychology/

The spectrum then moves on to how we might react normally in response to an abnormal event[15] like if we were involved in a car accident on the way to work or were suddenly called to the hospital to find a loved one in critical condition. In the trauma bay, I have seen people faint or become hysterical, even banging their heads on the floor after being told their loved one is grievously ill or injured. Such responses would be considered abnormal for normal conditions such as waking up or going to lunch, but are not necessarily abnormal for a crisis that has intruded into their otherwise normal day.

From there the spectrum moves on to abnormal responses in abnormal events, or in other words, reacting abnormally in the context of an abnormal occurrence. A good example of an abnormal response to an abnormal situation is one in which a man purposefully cut off his hand with a circular saw after having a fight with his parents. He lay stoically on the trauma bed as if he had not a care in the world as he watched the medical team work to save his arm. A normal response to the abnormal event of fighting with one's parents would be to get upset and maybe cry or storm off — not cut off one's hand.

Finally the spectrum moves towards abnormal responses to normal events. This can be seen in a soldier suffering with Post-Traumatic Stress Disorder (PTSD) who hears a noise in his sleep at home, imagines himself back on the battlefield fighting for his life, and wakes up to find himself strangling his wife who was sleeping next to him.

Psychiatry, in a medical setting, is focused on identifying, diagnosing, intervening, and caring for those who have developed abnormal reactions to both abnormal and normal situations. This often means dealing with patients with PTSD, drug and alcohol abuse problems, psychotic episodes, and so on.

---

15. Myers, D., & Wee, D.F. (2005). *Disaster mental Health services* (p. 26) New York, NY: Routledg Taylor & Francis Group.

Chaplaincy, contrastingly, is focused more on the opposite end of the spectrum, where we care for and manage patients with normal reactions during normal and abnormal life events.

In short, psychiatry is focused on abnormal responses and chaplaincy is focused on normal responses. This does not mean that one cannot recognize and handle the other end of the spectrum, but that caregivers from either group have a different starting point when it comes to care. One is looking for the abnormal and chaplains are looking for what is normal even in abnormal situations.

The implications of this are profound. For instance:

> *"About 6 of every 10 men (or 60%) and 5 of every 10 women (or 50%) experience at least one trauma in their lives. Women are more likely to experience sexual assault and child sexual abuse. Men are more likely to experience accidents, physical assault, combat, disaster, or to witness death or injury,"and yet only "…7 or 8 out of every 100 people (or 7-8% of the population) will have PTSD at some point in their lives."*[16]

This means that chaplaincy and the similar growing field of Critical Incidence Stress Management (CISM)[17] which also seeks to help people in natural and man-made disasters beyond chaplaincy, have the opportunity to intervene in the greatest number of people's lives, help them face the initial crisis that has caused a normal reaction to their abnormal situation, and help them to walk through the crisis, and find a normal life after the crisis has ended. This helps quell their normal reaction and calm them as the situation subsides before their reaction becomes prolonged and evolves into what could be classified as an abnormal response to what is now a

---

16. US Department of Veterans Affairs, PTSD: National Center for PTSD. How common is PTSD?. Retrieved from https://www.ptsd.va.gov/public/PTSD-overview/basics/how-common-is-ptsd.asp
17. Everly, G.S. Jr & Mitchell,J.T. (1997). *Critical incident stress management - A new era and standard of care in crisis intervention*. Ellicott City, MD: Chevron Publishing Corporation.

normal life requiring professional psychological help beyond chaplaincy (such would be the case for someone who has developed PTSD).

In other words, chaplains help shorten the time and potentially growing intensity of normal reactions to abnormal events and help prevent them from becoming long-term responses that might become PTSD or aggravate some other psychological problem.

Therefore, in general, it can be said that chaplaincy works with what is normal and psychiatry works with what has become a long-term abnormality.

It also means that chaplaincy and psychiatry need to work together. Even when a person has a psychological disorder, they still continue to experience normal reactions to abnormal situations/crisis beyond their disorder. A bipolar patient still often experiences normal grief if their parent dies and they need to be reassured that their feelings are normal and not necessarily part of their disorder. The relief on the face of a psychiatric patient has always amazed me when they realize that their grief is normal and not a part of the reason they were hospitalized.

The relief experienced, even by patients in the psych units I served, when recognizing what they were feeling or how they were thinking was not far different than what I might feel or think if I were in their shoes, was surprising to me as I began to care for people as a chaplain. The more I work with people, the broader my view of what is normal has become.

[illegible] and psychological [illegible] someone who [illegible]

[illegible] between the time and [illegible] abnormal events and [illegible] through [illegible] psychological problem.

[illegible] In general, it can be said that [illegible] that has become [illegible]

[illegible] and psychology [illegible] psychological [illegible] abnormal [illegible]

[illegible]

Chapter 2

Identifying What is 'Normal' in 'Abnormal' Situations

When we enter an abnormal crisis situation, how do we know if something is really an expected, normal reaction for an individual in that situation or the result of a mental illness that contributes to frequent abnormal responses?

The best way I can illustrate the answer is with how the FBI and Secret Service train their agents on how to spot counterfeit money. One agent has said that they were trained by studying only the real thing.[18] Instead of studying examples of what counterfeit money *could* look like, they spent their time learning every detail of real money.[19] The U.S. Currency Education Program is focused on the same thing.[20]

Likewise, chaplains learn about how to help people by learning what normal responses look like in both normal and abnormal situations. Then we seek to focus all of a person's resources in the best way possible by helping them manage their normal reactions to an abnormal crisis situation. We

18. Simons, S.G. (2008, January 1), Grace notes. Retrieved from http://www.e-gracenotes.org/article/2673/archives/the-bible-says/the-real-thing
19. How does the FBI train agents to spot counterfeit money? Retrieved from http://www.answers.com/Q/How_does_the_FBI_train_agents_to_spot_counterfeit_money?#slide=2
20. Dollars in detail. Retrieved from https://www.uscurrency.gov/sites/default/files/download-materials/en/CEP_Dollars_In_Detail_Brochure.pdf

also keep an eye on all those involved in a patient's care and help them realize when patients and their families are undergoing normal reactions to the present abnormal situation.

At the death of a parent, a child or adult is often told that they "have to be strong now for the family" and to stop crying. This normal response to the death of their mother or father is many times the cause of later psychological problems because they then try to hide their feelings to prevent themselves from crying. Much of my grief work with patients has been to give them permission to cry by teaching them and their families' that it often takes more strength to let others see how you are feeling than to hide those tearful feelings. It has also surprised me how often doctors and nurses try to equate being strong with not showing emotion since they often have to suppress how they are feeling at the moment in order to provide the care needed for their patient.

I remember a wife who, when told of the serious condition of her husband, slumped down unresponsive onto the floor of the family consult room. While I had been prepared for such a reaction because of our previous conversation, the nurse wasn't expecting it and called for a crash cart, thinking that the woman was having a heart attack. After making sure she was safely on the floor, I pointed out that the wife, though seemingly catatonic with a "thousand yard stare," was breathing in a normal fashion and not pale. The shock of the news had so overwhelmed her that she could not interact with the world around her for a time, but she was not having a heart attack. While the medical staff checked her out, I just sat on the floor with her and when she began to speak again she would only speak to me for a while, as she talked about her fears and what had happened. This can be a normal response to a situation not previously faced.

Initially her family became extremely angry, thinking that the staff had done something to her until I, in the midst of the event, reassured them that this can be a very normal initial reaction to shocking news. This helped avoid more emotion being added to the already stressful situation of the patient.

Chaplains are present to help everyone, family, friends, staff, and even patients, understand and work through what may be a very normal reaction to such an abnormal event/crisis, thus helping to avoid additional trauma from false ideas about what is happening. Family, friends, and even staff can easily become "secondary victims"[21] as they encounter and seek to help the person involved in a crisis.

A good place to add to one's understanding of what are normal reactions to an abnormal situation can be found in the U.S. Department of Veterans Affairs website, under their public PTSD section which contains a listing of common reactions faced by people in crisis.[22]

While well-intentioned, without proper expertise, one could easily mismanage the normal reaction of a person and only further hinder the recovery process for everyone involved in an abnormal situation.

---

21. Myers, D, & Wee, D. F. (2005), *Disaster Mental Health Services* (p.12). New York/London, NY/England: Routledge Taylor & Francis Group.
22. US Department of Veterans Affairs, PTSD: National Center for PTSD. Common reactions after trauma. Retrieved from https://www.ptsd.va.gov/public/problems/common-reactions-after-trauma.asp

Chapter 3

The Importance of Expertise

Everyone who is involved in a patient's care is there because of their expertise. The expertise of a care-provider is the easiest way to quantify and explain the value of that worker. To be quantified it must first be defined in ways that are understandable and valuable to others outside of that area of expertise.

In a 911 call, Emergency Medical Specialists (EMS) arrive on a scene because they are best trained in providing initial assessment, care, and timely transportation in medical emergencies.

Emergency doctors then provide care when patients are first brought into a hospital because their expertise is knowing how the body responds initially to a physical crisis.

As needed, other specialists such as orthopedics/cardiac/social work/chaplains are called in because of their ability to know and focus on specific areas of need. Meanwhile the emergency room doctors continue to focus on getting the patient stabilized to the point where the body can be able to begin its normal healing processes.

No one would ever say that an emergency room doctor does not know about mental/emotional/spiritual care of a patient or their family, but they would be the first to say they are not the absolute experts in those fields. Therefore, they call in the orthopedic doctors for broken bones, psychiatrists for attempted suicide or drug overdoses, chaplains for telling families/

patients what has happened, and so on for specific patient and family needs.

Chaplains focus in on their expertise even though possibly trained in other fields as well. One of my chaplain residency cohorts was a trained surgeon but would always call for the patient's doctor or psychiatrist or nurse when seeing something medical that needed to be done, letting them diagnose and treat that need. Likewise, I have always sought to include the entire medical team in my understanding of what might be going on with a patient and their family and sharing how that might impact their care. I also seek out the expertise of the other team members, seeking to learn from and honor their expertise.

How can we reasonably expect others to honor and listen to our expertise if we do not honor and listen to theirs?

An expert is considered such for a reason: they have more expertise in that area than others. They have an ability to sense the needs of a situation and ways of meeting those needs faster and better than other caregivers might. These heightened abilities in specific situations come from greater training and focused experience in specific fields.

When I was the trauma/emergency room chaplain for six years, I knew better than any of the other chaplains what to expect when a trauma patient arrived. When I eventually went on to perform other duties, I realized I would lose some of my touch with that type of patient. The chaplain who took over those duties in the ER would eventually become experienced in managing that style of care as I had. And when I moved on to another type of patient care, I gained a different type of expertise in palliative and intensive care.

Chaplaincy is a vital part of the medical team because of its expertise.

The EMS, doctors, nurses, specialists, and techs are part of the medical team because of their expertise in the physical and medical care of a person in crisis. They understand, diagnose, and intervene in the biological processes that have been damaged by trauma or illness.

Psychiatrists and psychologists are part of the medical team because of their expertise in the mental and emotional side of a person in crisis. They understand, diagnose, and intervene in the processes that have created long-term mental and emotional problems, causing people to not be able to care for themselves and/or others.

But what about chaplains? Why are they a vital part of a medical team and not just a luxury member of the team?

The language found in defining a chaplain's expertise

Developing the understanding of chaplaincy's impact on healthcare requires the ability to define our expertise and value to as many different types of people as possible in terms they can all easily understand and appreciate. This means finding words/concepts that are equally important and used consistently in all of these groups of people.

As I read the literature of doctors, researchers, nurses, social workers, pastors, administrators, and the public at large, there is one very personal word used consistently that speaks to the deepest convictions of most every person. Whether you are a patient, family, or staff, with either no education or many degrees, one word is consistently used by all. This word has a global concept that is less likely to be misunderstood; upon it all other chaplaincy concepts might be hung, taught, explained, and further developed: "belief."

Though much time is spent trying to define and refine the idea of chaplaincy in relationship to the caring of a person's "spiritual"[23] side, this lan-

23. Lichter, D.A. & O'Gorman, M.L. (2009, May-June). Establishing a chaplain's value. Retrieved from https://www.chausa.org/pastoralcare/resources/pastoral-care-articles/may-june-2009/establishing-a-chaplain's-value

guage seems to confuse or confine understanding more than clarify, as there is no clear consensus about what the 'spiritual' side of a person decidedly is. Some see it simply as the religious ideals of a person, while others argue that it is something more than a person's standard religious beliefs.[24]

Doctors and nurses usually call for a chaplain when a patient is dying or when a family is frustrated or bereft so that the chaplain may provide additional help to families, or perform requested religious rituals and services.

I was once called to help the adopted son of a woman who was expected to die within a few days. The son was angry that the nursing staff would not allow something he had requested. He loved his adoptive mother very much and had committed himself to her Christian faith. Even still, as he grew into adulthood he began to research and appreciate his Native American heritage. His adoptive mother always encouraged him to express his heritage, and he combined his traditional heritage with his and his mother's Christian faith. Traditionally, when someone in his tribe died, a candle or flame is lit to hold the dead person's soul for the duration of the person's funeral. At the end of the service, the flame is blown out and their soul released into the universe. He had brought a small chimney lantern to the hospital and asked if he could light the small flame when his mother died.

Needless to say, this was out of the question, as hospital policy would not allow for any open flame for safety reasons. That was why chaplains could provide only electric Shabbat candles for Jewish patients who asked for them.

This policy was deeply troubling to the son because his adoptive mother had so encouraged him to honor his heritage, and he had been planning this one ritual, beyond his Christian prayers, for a long time to honor his mother in death.

---

24. Hall, E.J., Hughes B.P., Handzo, G.H. (2016, October). *Spiritual care: what it means, why it matters in health care. Retrieved from* https://www.healthcarechaplaincy.org/docs/about/spirituality.pdf

After listening to his story and seeing her rapidly deteriorating condition, I went to the nursing supervisor and got her to check with the safety officer of the hospital in order to get permission for this request.

Because of a chaplain's involvement in the situation, an exception to the hospital's policy was made with safety precautions put in place to allow for the lighting of the lamp.

She died that night, and the flame was lit and taken by a grateful son soon thereafter.

Chaplains deal with situations like these consistently. While hospital staff usually think to call upon a chaplain when death or unusual religious rituals are desired, they often do not think to involve us when family is being told of a negative diagnosis or when hard decisions need to be made. A chaplain might be called to observe and aid a Shaman with rocks, feathers, and bones or Muslim family wanting to wash their loved one's dead body, but we are there for more than just religious rituals or activities.

Chaplains' duties beyond those of religious support are becoming a greater aspect of our duties as our society sees themselves more as "spiritual" and less traditionally "religious." There is a growing percentage of the population that identifies as atheists, agnostics, and those who claim no religious affiliation and as a result, the importance and requirements of chaplaincy is shifting.

A recent Pew research survey determined that 23 percent of the U.S. population classifies themselves as "nones," or those who might fall under a type of "non-religious" categories. This number is up from 16 percent of the population just seven years prior.[25] 37 percent of Americans claim to be "spiritual" as opposed to "religious."[26]

---

25. Lipka, M. (2015/05/13), A closer look at America's rapidly growing religious 'nones'. Retrievedfromhttp://pewresearch.org/fact-tank/2015/05/13/a-closer-look-at-american-rapidely-growing-religious-nones
26. Pew Research Center (2012, October 9). Retrieved from http://www.pewforum.org/2012/10/09/nones-on-the-rise

With the ever increasing levels of diversity in our society, the way we communicate has become more and more fragmented and excluding. As religious terminology becomes less understood by society at large, there becomes a greater need to find simplified concepts that can unify our understandings while still allowing for diversity. Words and phrases that are used to describe spirituality become too technical at times and their meaning is lost or misunderstood across the different social groups. Terms and phrases used to define spirituality like "intrinsic," "ultimate meaning," "transcendence," "relationship to self," "impaired ability to experience and integrate meaning and purpose in life," and "connectedness" all require a level of technical knowledge that has different meanings for different people.

These words and phrases are commonly understood between chaplains seeking to define spirituality to other chaplains as in Healthcare Chaplaincy Network's 2016 article, "Spiritual Care: What It Means, Why It Matters in Health Care,"[27] but little meaning to others outside the institution.

For instance: the idea of "connectedness" to chaplains speaks of interacting on a personal level, while to a doctor it might primarily carry a sense of interacting on a professional level, and to an IT person it speaks of electronic connectivity.

While it is good to more deeply explore concepts in greater technical terms, there is a need to ultimately simplify not only one's understanding around a few more commonly held concepts, but also to help others better understand the situation.

Therefore, let's look at the chaplain's expertise and seek to simplify the concept of "spiritual" care with a more commonly understood word. That way we have a concept to which all other chaplaincy ideas may be easily attached.

---

27. Hall, E. J., Hughes, B. P. & Handzo, G. H. (2016, October). Retrieved from https://www.healthcarechaplaincy.org/docs/about/spirituality.pdf

As we have already discussed, the medical staff's expertise lies in the biological and physical processes of the patient, the psychologists work with mental and emotional faculties, and the chaplains care for the spiritual side of recovery (See Figure 2).

MEDICAL TEAM MEMBERS EXPERTISE

Doctors, Nurses, EMTs –

Biological processes, i.e. physical side

Psychiatrists & Psychologists –

Mental & Emotional processes, i.e. thinking and feeling side

Chaplains –

Belief processes, i.e. spiritual side

(Figure 2)

"I/we believe"[28] and "people believe" are one of the most common refrains used in the writings of all categories of society. From the pastor, to the doctor, to the researcher, to care givers, and administrators, as well as patients and their families, everyone acts based on their perception of what is true, which is a part of belief.

> *"Norris et al. found that the disaster research findings were very consistent regarding the benefits of one's beliefs about one's own ability to cope. That is, what matters is not how individuals actually cope, but rather how they perceive their abilities to cope and control outcomes . . .*

28. Everly, G.S. Jr. & Mitchell, J.F. (2008). *Integrative crisis intervention and disaster mental health.* Ellicott City, MD: Chevron Publishing Corporation.

> *The perception that one can cope is strongly predictive of good psychological outcomes (Benight, Ironson, et al., 1999; Benight, Swift, Sanger, Smith, & zeppelin, 1999[29]).*"[30]

Chaplains provide a greater expertise to the medical team beyond just the impact of a patient's religious beliefs. They also work with the impact of a patient's/family's/friend's beliefs about doctors, medicine, and their families, which becomes even more valuable in the palliative care aspects of medical care. The importance of belief can be seen in many palliative care studies carried on in recent years like in "Approaching Patients and Family Members Who Hope for a Miracle."[31]

Chaplaincy is a vital part of the medical team because of its important "expertise." This importance, I have found, is best expressed in the language of the "expertise" of "belief processes", which makes chaplains a vital, needed part of the medical team and more easily understood by all parties involved when providing care to a patient.

Whether providing religious counsel or helping a patient and family face their beliefs about the hospital, doctors, medicine, etc., a chaplain must use the best language possible, whether using the language of words, the language of deeds, or even the language of appropriate silence.

---

29. Benight, C., Swift, E., Sanhger, J., Smith, A., & Zeppelin, D. (1999). Coping self-efficacy as a mediator of distress following a natural disaster. Journal of Applied Social Psychology, 29, 2443-2464.
30. .Benight, C., Swift, E., Sanhger, J., Smith, A., & Zeppelin, D. (1999). Coping self-efficacy as a mediator of distress following a natural disaster. Journal of Applied Social Psychology, 29, 2443-2464.
31. Fromme, E.K. & Arnold, R.M. (2011), Approaching patients and family members who hope for a miracle, *Journal of Pain and Symptom Management*, Abstract. Retrieved from http://www.jpsmjournal.com/article/S0885-3924(11)00243-0/fulltext

Chapter 4

Working Tangibly with the Spiritual Side of a Patient

The spiritual side of a person is where perceived truth and emotion merge.

Belief is not just a group of perceived truths, thoughts, ideas; it is where thoughts and feelings merge. A belief is grown and held only when a perceived truth becomes tied to emotion.

I and my twin brother used to argue about many things. Often we took opposite sides, not because of our beliefs but simply because we liked to argue and see who was better at it. We took on a possible truth without having any other personal emotion tied to it than that of not wanting the other to be seen as having a better argument.

A true belief holds not only perceived truth but deep emotional attachment as well.

All you have to do is watch a person in church singing about a great truth of their faith with tears running down their cheek to realize that belief involves not just ideas but ideas that have become tied to deep emotion. Where and how that merging takes place is the spiritual side of a person.

Another example are protesters as they not only carry signs and chant slogans but also those who torch cars and face off with those who disagree with them, to know, that their beliefs carry great ideas tied to great emotion, right or wrong, for good or ill.

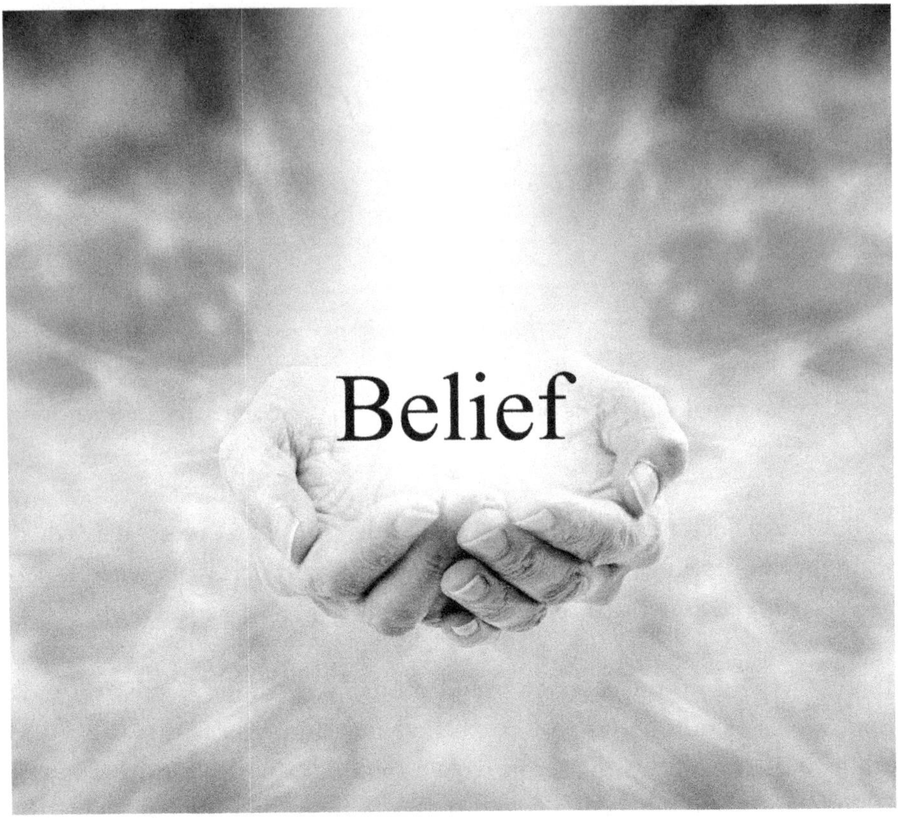

The belief/spiritual side of a person…

Finds and gives meaning to life and events: The 'perceived truth' part of belief

Helping people find meaning in the midst of crisis is a basic element of being a chaplain. This is such a key concept that even chaplaincy organizations like the Healthcare Chaplaincy Network use it in the initial description of themselves: "Healthcare Chaplaincy Network is a nonprofit health care organization that helps people faced with distress and illness and suffering to find comfort and meaning."[32] (Notice that "comfort", a feeling, is tied to "meaning", a perception.)

For some, belief begins with an idea that evolves and attaches to emotions, transforming it from a belief into a "conviction." These convictions are organized in our lives in ways that bring about order and congruence. A person with convictions often willfully ignores information that does not affirm ideas in which they believe; in psychology, this exclusion of conflicting ideas is called cognitive dissonance. An example of this would be a family member who refuses to acknowledge a patient's deteriorating health because their loved one is too precious to die and their failing health does not fit into their perception of the wonders of modern medicine.

Reaches out to something beyond themselves: Believing in Some*thing*

Whenever we reach out to touch anything in this world we are involving ourselves in a spiritual/belief activity. When we sit in a chair, it is a type of spiritual activity. We look at the chair in order to evaluate that it can hold us and then we have to emotionally relax into that chair in order to truly believe that it will support our weight.

Connects with someone beyond themselves: Believing in Some*one*

One of the most important duties of a chaplain is to connect with others.

When we connect with another person, it is a spiritual/belief activity because we must first perceive that it is safe to interact. The desire for connection is needed to create the belief that the interaction will be positive enough to make the effort worth experiencing.

32. Healthcare Chaplaincy Network. Retrieved from https://healthcarechaplaincy.org/clinical-pastoral-education.html

Then one must develop a feeling of closeness in order to feel safe enough to interact on deeper levels.

The ultimate relationship and interaction for many is their relationship with God.

Creates hope: Believing in a future

Much of chaplaincy involves the acquisition, development, continuation, and refocusing of hope. Many books having been written just on this topic, such as Michael W. and Kathy J. Langstrom's "A Journey to Hope – Healing the Traumatized Spirit."[33]

Hope can be seen as the perception that a certain activity will result in a good outcome merged with the emotion of anticipating a positive future.

Drives their choices: The results of belief

When we insist that something we perceive is the truth, we engage in a mental activity. When this perceived truth ties itself to an emotion, we engage in a spiritual activity. It then becomes a belief, whether positive or negative. It is not just in solely the mental activity or solely the emotional activity that a chaplain's expertise lies, but in the understanding of the merging of perceived truth and emotion as one experience. How does this convergence happen? What are its effects? How can we best intervene and interact, without stepping on the other's autonomy? It is in these roles that the function and value of chaplaincy lie.

How do perceived truths and emotions merge?

First, we need to remember that all people, when confronted with trauma or crisis, respond first from one of two places: mentally or emotionally.

33. Langstrom, M. W. & Langstrom, K. J. (2016). *A journey to hope – healing the traumatized spirit.* Silverton, OR: Lampion Press.

If there is a fire in an apartment building and someone comes running out to the fire trucks as they arrive, they will approach those arriving in one of two ways. They might efficiently explain everyone had gotten out of the building except for one family who did not come to the door. Or, they could come out so flustered and terrified that they are incoherent for a while, unable to arrange their thoughts.

I have seen parents immediately begin planning and making decisions about who needed to be called and what needed to be done when they had been told their child died. Others have fallen to the floor unable to speak through their tears. Both were expressing their sense of loss from their personal starting point. Neither is wrong in their reaction; they simply have different ways of beginning to process a crisis or trauma.

The one who started from a logical, more analytical place surely also had a great emotional response, but had to first work through their initial thoughts and reaction before they could face their emotions. Conversely, the one who started from an emotional place needed to first work through their initial feelings, before being able to organize their thoughts logically.

We all start from one side or the other. Thoughts and feelings are not mutually exclusive to themselves or to any situation. We all have both. The difference lies in what we personally begin to process first.

This is why chaplains need to be versed in caring for people in crisis on both levels: logical and emotional. A chaplain must be ready to face either initial reaction and help them work through it to get to the other. They must be able to move back and forth between thoughts and feelings as a person processes a given situation. Furthermore, a chaplain must be able to move quickly between reactions, back and forth with an individual as they fluctuate between thoughts and feelings, multiplied by other family members facing their own crisis, each at different points in their processes and reactions.

These two main types of response continue to be studied, but a new emphasis has been placed on the importance of working with the emotional side of a person. Dr. Travis Bradberry, who studies the performance of people in everyday jobs, has emphasized the need for "emotional intelligence" in workers and managers in the everyday workplace because he has found that people with average intelligence outperformed people with high IQs 70 percent of the time in their management and work duties.[34] Dr. Bradberry has developed ways to quantify emotional aptitude and strengthen a person's 'emotional quotient' or "EQ"[35], as he calls it. By doing this, he hopes to help people become better managers and workers.

The process of merging perceived truth with emotions normally happens when a person experiences a crisis in relationship to him or herself, another, or God. Relationships between two individuals or to oneself are normally the catalyst, for good or ill, of the merging of a perceived truth with an emotion.

Many people have told me that they have been attracted to the churches I pastored because of the connections and relationships they had made with other congregants.

Many have also said that they have been attracted to other churches or religions, like the Mormon Church for instance, because of the strong emphasis on family relationships within the church. People often change their ideals and beliefs based on their relationships and how something affects those relationships.

It is out of the need for relationships that changes in belief usually happen.

34. Bradberry, T. (2015, January 7). Why you need emotional intelligence. Retrieved from https://www.forbes.com/sites/travisbradberry/2015/01/07/why-you-need-emotional-intelligence-to-succeed/#7574ffda6246/

35. Bradberry, T. & Greaves, J. (2015) Emotional intelligence 2.0. Retrieved from http://www.talentsmart.com/products/emotional-intelligence-2.0/

Chapter 5

What is the purpose of chaplaincy involvement?

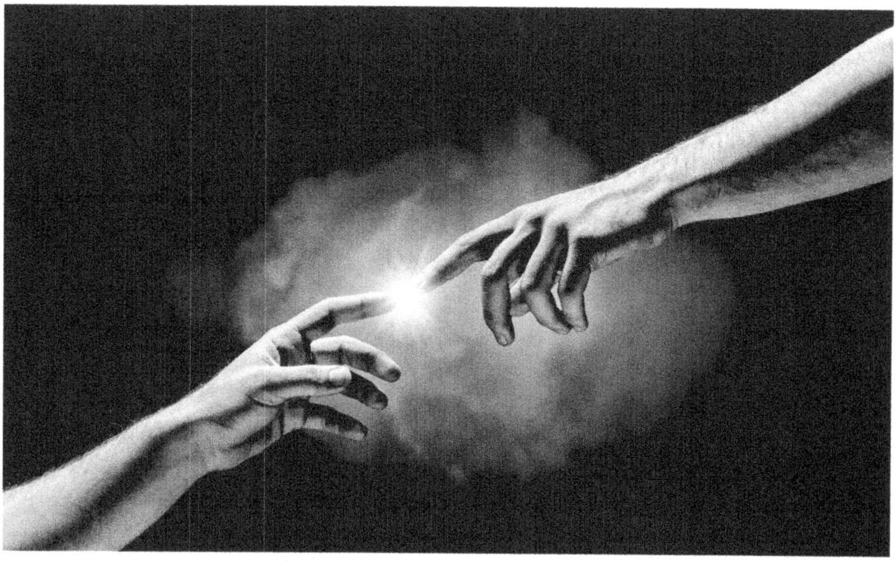

A chaplain's expertise is in the personal belief processes of people. We intervene without stepping on the autonomy of the other and help them work through their reactions to crises. We help them integrate their beliefs, whatever they may be, into their recovery process by making their thoughts and feelings more congruent with each other. We do this so that they might make better choices than they might have originally without help.

In a medical setting, while diagnosing, treating, and caring for someone, we ask people to make choices. These choices need to be ones that they will not regret later on upon retrospect. From allowing themselves to be taken to the hospital via ambulance, to putting in IVs, to cutting off all of their clothes in the trauma bay and allowing tests be done for diagnosis and treatment, choices have to be made and they have to be made with full conviction.

Making choices and compliance

Ultimately, compliance, which affects much of modern medicine's ability to provide quality care, rests with a patient and their family's choices.

Compliance only truly comes when choices are made with conviction out of personal beliefs. If manipulated into a choice, or directed by the force of another's personality, a person will back out or not follow through with the choice as soon as they are no longer feeling coerced. If a person chooses something without having been provided the opportunity to allow personal emotion to become tied to it (which often takes time), the choice likely will not last. It will be a choice without conviction and, therefore, without compliance.

This is why, so often, patients will set up appointments and not keep them; why patients will take a prescription from a doctor but not fill it; why so many patients come back into the hospital in under 30 days with further complications. Such instances forced most hospitals in 2016 to bear a 3 percent penalty for such readmissions from Medicare.[36]

36. Rice, S. (2015). Most hospitals face 30-day readmissions penalty in fiscal 2016. *Modern healthcare* http://www.modernhealthcare.com/article/20150803/NEWS/150809981/

The interplay of choices, belief, and "patient-centered" care

The new watchword of healthcare is that of patient-centered care. "This once radical concept has undeniably been pushed into the mainstream."[37] Patient-centered care must start with a patient's beliefs about what is happening to them and grow into an understanding of what they believe will help.

If belief is the foundation of all choices and patient-centeredness is considered foundational for quality and patient safety in today's medical care,[38] then patient-centeredness requires the understanding of a patient's beliefs as a foundational process to caring for the patient and their families in the best way.

This is not just limited to what a person believes about God and religious spirituality, but also what they believe about their situation, doctors, medicine, and their family/friends who claim to be helping them.

If a patient believes that God will intervene and perform a miracle to heal them, they are unlikely to follow medical advice or discuss options that do not adhere to their expectation of an imminent miracle.

I once overheard a doctor explaining to a family why a Do Not Resuscitate (DNR) order might be the best for their loved one. She did a wonderful job explaining the situation, the available options, and what they were doing to try to help. The family listened intently to the doctor until she began to approach the idea of a DNR. She suggested the order because it is often a good option when age and non-responsiveness to treatments are a factor. After being cut off in shock and anger by the family, the doctor took a deep breath and began again to try to encourage the DNR from a different ap-

37. Frampton, S., Guastello S., Brady, C., Hale, M., Horowitz, S. Smith, S.B. & Stone S. *(2008). Patient-centered care improvement guide (*p. 3) Patient-Centered Care.org
38. Frampton, S., Guastello S., Brady, C., Hale, M., Horowitz, S. Smith, S.B. & Stone S. *(2008). Patient-centered care improvement guide (*p. 3) Patient-Centered Care.org

proach. Again, the family cut her off, aghast at the mere suggestion. A third time the doctor tried to explain the benefit of a DNR and again the family cut her off. Frustrated, she turned on her heels and left them without saying another word. I stayed around and talked with them, and eventually found out that they believed God was going to heal their grandmother. Therefore, entertaining even the idea of a DNR was unnecessary and would be considered a lack of faith in God.

If a person stalwartly believes that their doctor only wants to perform surgery on them because he wants a new swimming pool in his backyard, the patient is not likely to agree to the surgery, regardless of how much the medical team insists.

If a person does not believe in taking pills, they will have a harder time being compliant with required medication. Contrastingly, if they believe that medicine is the ultimate answer, they might think that taking a double dose will heal them twice as fast.

If a person believes that another family member does not have their best interest in mind, they will make choices that are contrary to what that family member and the doctor both believe would be best. I once knew a man who insisted on leaving the hospital even though he was in need of a major surgery, all because he did not trust his family members living in his house.

All these beliefs can interfere with what is best for the patient. To allow for patient-centered care, you must know and understand what beliefs enable and inhibit patient-centered care and how to intervene in those beliefs without stepping on the autonomy of the other.

Chaplains have to help the entire medical team understand the patient's point of view and how it is impacting their relationship to the team.

Chapter 6

Where does the need for chaplains come from?

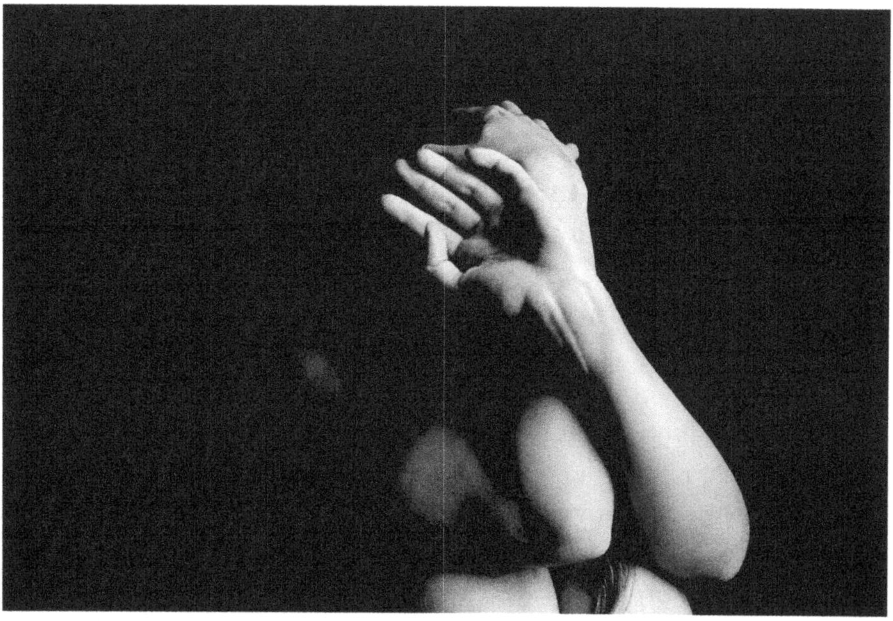

The challenge a crisis places on belief

In a crisis a person is often stripped of the masks and walls that we put up to protect our inner selves from the outside world. These defenses are perceptions, good and bad, that affect not only how others might see us but also how we see ourselves.

People can become very fearful and angry when others are able to see them as they really are, stripped bare of their defenses. They fear that people, seeing them unsure, weak, or emotional, will take advantage of them or judge them harshly. Crisis has a way of revealing how we really think and feel. It can bring out the best or the worst in people.

Crises or "critical incidents" as George Everly and Jeffrey Mitchell put it, "are stressful events which have the potential to overwhelm one's usual coping mechanisms resulting in psychological distress and an impairment of normal individual, as well as collective, adaptive functioning."[39] When "overwhelmed" a person does not have the energy to keep up their protective psychological walls anymore.

So, upon hearing that a mother/grandmother had died, the daughter and granddaughter of the deceased began to immediately argue, in my presence, about who would possess the lottery tickets that their mother/grandmother had just purchased that day. The argument quickly devolved and the granddaughter, shortly followed thereafter by the daughter, ran out of the room to get home and get the lottery tickets before the other.

Crisis draws out the true nature of people, and not everyone likes what they see, from the individuals themselves to those around them.

A girl was once brought into the trauma bay who had just tried to commit suicide by jumping off the third story of a building. As I sat with her, she spoke about getting ready to graduate from nursing school that same day. I was confused by the inconsistency between the joy of graduation resulting in trying to commit suicide. It eventually came out that she had been telling her family that she had been going to nursing school and the graduation was that day, but that none of it was true. Fearing what her family would think of her when the truth came out, she jumped. By the time the

39. Everly, G.S. Jr, & Mitchell, J.T. (1997). *Critical incident stress management, a new era and standard of care in crisis intervention* (p. 4). Ellicott City, MD: Chevron Publishing Corporation.

family arrived at the ICU, the hospital had already been told by the nursing school that there was no record of her ever having attended there.

The girl had finally begun to own up to the lies she had been telling her family by admitting to me the true situation. Yet, when the family arrived, the girl was again telling her family that she had been on the way to graduation and did not know why she had jumped. The family's presence had drawn her back into the tale of her working to become a nurse. With them looking down at her in intensive care, she could not help but return to her lies, which were more palatable to her than the truth.

When, during crises, our masks and coping mechanisms are often stripped away, we find ourselves to be at our most vulnerable. These masks can be of our own making or masks that have been made because of the expectations of others. I have often heard one family member tell another family member to "be strong and stop crying" when told of a death or injury, as if revealing how they truly felt was a bad thing or a weakness to be hidden. The stopping of needed emotional expression is a type of injury that can be inflicted when a wall is stripped away during a crisis.

This is why chaplains enter every situation with great care, seeking to understand the lives/beliefs of everyone involved, without casting judgment or injury. A wife, who just lost her husband, may find great support in her faith, while their child might seek to seemingly comfort their mother with platitudes like, "he's in a better place" but are meanwhile effectively avoiding their own pain and emotion that needs to be felt and accepted.

This vulnerability often comes from being confronted with the inconsistencies in our beliefs that become more apparent when our masks are removed by the stress of a crisis.

One aspect of being human is that we can often hold two opposing beliefs simultaneously without knowing it. We can act in a way contrary to our beliefs or have feelings that seem contrary to our beliefs. This incongruence is at the root of much of what psychology seeks to correct.

For example, I might believe that God is in control of everything that happens to me but, at the same time, try to control my surroundings, feeling that I cannot trust anyone, including God.

This incongruence between our thinking and actual emotion tied to that perceived truth is often what makes us build masks and make choices that seem out of place or inconsistent themselves. This incongruence is a basic feature of human beings and the key element chaplains work to identify and help modify so people will be more willing and able to make better choices, choices that they will be less likely to regret in the future. I write more about this later in the religious/Biblical reflection on belief.

In a crisis, a person is confronted with their fears (real or imagined). This is especially true of a medical crisis. Fears are based on one's beliefs about life and death, life becoming more limited, or the uncertainty of life.

How often has a parent, when told that their son or daughter has been shot, asked the question, "Are they dead?"

Very often a person is confronted with the realization that they do not know what they actually believe in and/or how they feel, and therefore he/she need time to process both their thoughts and feelings.

We live in a society that has lost much of its ability to stop, in the midst of life, and reflect on inner thoughts and emotions, i.e. our beliefs. The hectic pace of society and the desire to get ahead does not allow much time to stop and reflect on our inner selves.

Also, our own personal hesitancy to discover and look at our thoughts and feelings which would show us the incongruences and inadequacies in our life causes us to avoid facing the reality of what we believe.

This has led to the rise of "life coaches" as fewer numbers in our society choose to turn to religion and the support of a congregation. Religion is a place to meditate on life and death, yet fewer and fewer people are aligning themselves with religious thought.

Remember the Pew Research study published in 2015 referred to earlier? One of its summary statements was, "The Christian share of the U.S. population is declining, while the number of U.S. adults who do not identify with any organized religion is growing, according to an extensive new survey by the Pew Research Center" published in 2015.[40]

As chaplains, our focus is to help patients discover and have conviction in their beliefs, by being with them in person and in support of their beliefs. By helping them along the way during a crisis, those convictions and beliefs are, hopefully, less wavering in the face of stress and crisis.

The effects of belief's control of choices for chaplains

Choices need to be understood and in line with a person's beliefs (not just religious beliefs). If we do not discover, explore, and tie the choices being requested to a person's beliefs in the patient's, family's, care giver's, manager's, administrators', clergy's thinking, we lose one of the greatest opportunities to collectively impact the patient's care and express clearly what chaplains' work is about. When everyone is on the same page they can bring their own individual expertise to the situation, with a common language that creates common goals to help people feel supported and not give mixed messages as a medical team.

A person's beliefs can help or hurt them when facing life's uncertainties. What one believes causes a person to join hands with another when facing a crisis or shove the other's hand away. It draws us into accepting or rejecting help.

If I believe you are there to help me and have my best interests in mind, I will hear what you are saying and more openly consider what you are suggesting. If I believe you are only interested in protecting yourself or pro-

40. Pew Research Center. (2015 May 12). America's changing religious landscape. Retrieved from http://www.pewforum.org/2015/05/12/americas-changing-religious-landscape/

moting your own interests, I will more likely misunderstand what you are saying and reject what is being suggested.

One of the chaplain's greatest values to the medical team is their ability to discover, explore, and engage another's beliefs and make sure the entire team understands the impact of those beliefs on their decisions and reactions to the crisis at hand. We act as interpreters for both sides, using the patient's beliefs as a language. This provides a common avenue from which to approach a situation so that patients and families do not feel like they are getting different stories from different providers.

The family of a comatose person can often feel confused if one specialist, like a kidney doctor, says that the patient's kidneys are doing better but the neurologist comes in saying that the brain is herniating and the patient is dying. The family, wishing for a cure, hears the doctor saying the kidneys are doing better, and interprets that as 'the patient is doing better.' Not wanting to believe that their loved one is dying, the family rejects what the neurologist is saying and strikes out in anger at the patient's nurse when he says the patient is not doing well. In this scenario it would be better for the kidney doctor to identify not only the kidneys are doing better, but also that this will not change the fact that the brain is herniating and the patient's health is still declining.

The need to help people find their deepest beliefs

A chaplain greatly helps a patient and their family by helping them discover, evaluate, and make conscious choices about what their deepest beliefs are. If choices are understood and made out of a person's deepest beliefs, they are less likely to regret a choice made with the information at hand. Even if, in retrospect, a person would have made a different choice based on new information, the regret will be less because the basis of the choice at the time was a person's beliefs which are made with conviction more than information that might later be revised.

Therefore, discovering and strengthening one's resolve about their deepest beliefs can help in making the difficult choices that are often a part of healthcare. This is true whether working with a patient, their family, or the medical team.

The effects of conflicting beliefs

Conflicting beliefs create inaction and "misaction."

We as human beings often hold two or more opposite beliefs at any one time, without even realizing it ourselves. However, when a crisis breaks down our walls and masks, these opposing beliefs become visible and wreak havoc. The incongruence creates inaction as we go back and forth between two different views, not knowing which belief to act upon. In the case of medical situations we become immobilized or not able to make a decision, which can have disastrous consequences.

If a family member believes that a loved one is not going to die because medicine can fix nearly everything, if applied soon enough, but also believe, more foundationally, that a person's life is controlled by God and it is His ultimate choice when one dies, they can fall into a spiraling crisis themselves of not being able to form convictions based on either belief. This is when a chaplain helps that person find their more foundational belief and bring it into focus. By doing so, this will help them accept a patient's death should it come, rather than blame the doctor for having done something wrong or, even worse, blame themselves for not being able to make a solid decision because they were spiraling and indecisive. This carries with it a huge impact on both the medical teams care and the administrator's bottom line, not to mention helps to ease the emotional weight on the patient and their loved ones.

It has always surprised me how many people actually believe that medicine undeniably will be able to completely solve their loved one's crisis. Families not only face disappointment by clinging to this false idea, but also place extraordinary responsibility upon the doctors and other medical personnel who can only do their best. Coming to the realization there is nothing more that can be done to save a loved one is hard for everyone. Because medicine can sometimes seem to produce miracles, we find it hard to accept the reality of there being limitations to what we can do as human beings with our knowledge base. That being said, when we remember our deepest convictions and beliefs and join hands in facing the realities of life's limitations together, we are able to make better choices for the sake of the patient in spite of a bad situation.

So many times, I have seen families and doctors push for continuing aggressive medical treatments even when there were no other effective treatments to offer. Their love and fear for the patient blinded them from reason. However, they almost all eventually faced the reality of human limitation and the futility of aggressive care when they remembered and took hold of their deepest beliefs which helped them look beyond medicine.

I define "misaction" as a choice that later is regretted or becomes a source of blame.

When we are pushed or are manipulated into a choice, we act against our beliefs, and in so doing create fertile ground to blame another for the choice we allowed to be made.

Choices that are not consciously made out of our deepest beliefs become the place from which blame grows and creates the unwillingness to accept responsibility for those choices.

Therefore, congruency of belief needs to be a focus when chaplains deal with people in medical situations. Until incongruence is faced and a realignment of personal beliefs are made, there is great potential for inaction or misaction and resulting strife.

How often are patients and families unwilling to make a choice about a needed surgery or other treatments? Rather than helping someone realign their beliefs and make decisions with conviction, often they choose to wait around for the decision-maker to sort it out for themselves. This is where a chaplain comes in to help.

The ultimate effect of belief

Ultimately, how we act on our beliefs connects or disconnects us from our resources. Belief is the starting point of all choices and who we choose to let help us when we're in need is dependent upon what we believe about them. We can only provide the quality of care that will be believed in by the patient and family. All other care will be either rejected, misunderstood, or blame filled, should it fail to improve the patient's health.

This effects the quality of care that can be provided by the medical team, hospitals, communities, and families.

Much of the effectiveness of a medical team's work is dependent upon the compliance of the patient, not only during a hospital stay but after they go home. Follow-up appointments, a regiment of medicine, needed change in lifestyle, and so on will all be ignored if a patient does not truly believe in the effectiveness of any one or all of them.

Compliance is dependent more on a person's beliefs than statistics, research, good arguments, or requirements; it is dependent on the choices we decide to make for ourselves based on our beliefs.

Chapter 7

What chaplains have learned from psychotherapy

The greatest contribution that psychology has made to a chaplain's expertise lies in the secularization of religious language into a more understandable common verbiage. While psychological terminology has created its own need for simplification over time, the various psychological specializations began with simple, easily understood concepts. Chaplains have used these various concepts to help others as they have integrated many of them with their own beliefs. Truth is still truth wherever it is found.

Talk therapy

When we think of modern psychology Sigmund Freud, who is considered the father of modern day psychological thought, is the first person to come to mind. He began with a focus on what he called "talk therapy."[41] Talk therapy is based on the idea that healing psychological problems can be accomplished through a non-directive, conversational interaction, making that which is unconscious become conscious.[42] While not all of Freud's theories may be helpful to chaplaincy development, you can definitely see his style in the way chaplains focus their healing interactions around con-

41. Wieman, R. (2015 July 7). Sigmund Freud (1856-1939). Retrieved from http://www.goodtherapy.org/famous-psychologists/sigmund-freud.html
42. History of psychotherapy. Retrieved from https://en.wikipedia.org/wiki/History_of_psychotherapy

versation. Part of chaplains' expertise is the ability to connect with others through "talk."

The therapeutic relationship

Positive change can come from a therapeutic relationship, so defining what a therapeutic relationship should look like is a key component of beginning to help. The concept of a therapeutic relationship began with Freud and continues to be studied by members of all fields of human care, but especially those in the healthcare field. Katarina Gadjanski BSc(Hons), LCCH, RSHom writes,

> *"The problem that we face within the medical profession in general is that the professional training provided to medical students (including homeopathy students and other health professionals) is not quite sufficient in teaching inter-personal and basic counseling skills which are invaluable therapeutic tools, and which are especially important when we want to create a successful therapeutic relationship with our patients... Unfortunately a lot of the medical schools do not stress this fact enough during the medical training. The doctors and medical practitioners in general are left to develop these inter-relational skills at their own discretion . . . Within my training I soon learnt that in psychotherapy the therapeutic relationship is, what Jung called,* "the alpha and the omega" *of the treatment . . . [and that] the relationship between a therapist and a client would play a crucial role in the treatment [of a patient] . . . However, I would argue that quality of the therapeutic relationship is as an important factor in other kinds of* 'helping' *relationships . . . The human mind and body are not split from each other and, therefore, physical pathology should not be seen and treated as something separate from the whole person. It would be of great value if the medical profession could adopt this approach from psychotherapy."*[43] *

43. Gadjanski, K, The importance of a therapeutic relationship - in psychotherapy and beyond. Retrieved from www.chiswickhomeopathyclinic.co.uk/TherapeuticRelationship.Artic..doc

*Direct quote edited for grammar and punctuation.

A chaplain's expertise contains an understanding of the therapeutic relationship with its implied abilities to connect quickly with others in non-directive ways. A chaplain seeks to have a person make choices without manipulating or necessarily having a specific choice being promoted.

Carl Rogers' four basic concepts

Humanistic psychologist Carl Rogers first created what he called "Client-Centered" therapy in which help is provided through a therapeutic relationship focusing on the client discovering for themselves what their need is and what answers might meet that need. Rogers' therapy centered on the idea that the patient is the expert about himself and the therapist is an expert in creating the kind of relationship that will provide a safe place for the patient to explore their own issues and answers.

Rogers' 'client-centered' therapy is a type of psychology with which modern chaplains most closely align their practices in medical situations today. Also, the idea of being client-centered parallels the strong, new focus upon which the government has placed medical care with its regulations that pay more to medical facilities that can show greater patient satisfaction.

Organizations like Planetree have grown out of the need that is now affecting a medical facilities bottom line.

> "*With the introduction of the HCAHPS (Hospital Consumer Assessment of Healthcare Providers and Systems) patient experience of care survey, there now exists a standardized tool to evaluate the way care is provided from the patient perspective. The program's development has reinforced that, from the vantage point of patients, the health care experience encompasses much more than clinical capabilities, pharmaceuticals, and technology. Whereas other nationally standardized and publicly reported outcomes . . . like CMS's core measures, evaluate hospitals on aspects of clinical quality, that mean little to patients themselves and/or reflect outcomes that patients take for granted as minimum standards of care, HCAHPS examines those aspects of the health care*

experience that mean the most to patients, including communication with nurses and physicians, cleanliness and noise levels, pain control, and quality of discharge instructions and medication information. With individual hospitals' scores publicly available for the curiosity, scrutiny, and comparability of health care consumers, HCAHPS has hastened the need for hospitals to examine the way care is delivered from the perspective of their patients. And with the advent of value-based purchasing, HCAHPS will likely become a basis for reimbursement, effectively advancing patient-centered care from the right thing to do to a business imperative."[44] *

Carl Rogers then builds his care with a focus on the therapeutic relationship based on three basic principles, Unconditional Positive Regard, Empathy, and Congruence.[45]

1. Unconditional positive regard is where a caregiver has an "outgoing, positive feeling, without reservations, without evaluations"[46] toward a patient and that "the more of this there is that therapy will be successful."[47*]

2. Empathy is "experiencing an accurate empathic understanding of the client's private world . . . To sense the client's inner world of private personal meanings as if it were your own, but without ever losing the 'as if' quality . . . To sense his anger or his fear or his feeling of being persecuted as if it were your own, and yet without your own anger, fear, or suspicion getting bound up in it."[48*]

---

44. Frampton, S., Guastello, S., Brody, C., Hale, M., Horowitz, S., Smith, S.B., Stone, S. (2008 October). *Patient improvement care improvement guide* (p.3). *Retrieved from* http://www.patient-centeredcare.org
45. Rogers, C. (1962 January 19). *The therapeutic relationship: Recent theory and research.* Beverly Hills, California: Los Angeles Society of Clinical Psychologists.
46. Rogers, C. (1962 January 19). *The therapeutic relationship: Recent theory and research* (p.4). Beverly Hills, California: Los Angeles Society of Clinical Psychologists.
47. Rogers, C. (1962 January 19). *The therapeutic relationship: Recent theory and research (p.4).* Beverly Hills, California: Los Angeles Society of Clinical Psychologists.
48. Rogers, C. (1962 January 19). *The therapeutic relationship: Recent theory and research (p5).* Beverly Hills, California: Los Angeles Society of Clinical Psychologists.

3. Congruence is "a therapist is what he is, when in the relationship with his client he is genuine and 'without front' or façade, openly being the feelings and attitudes which at that moment are flowing in him . . . that the feelings the therapist is experiencing are available to him, available to his awareness, that he is able to live these feelings, be them, and able to communicate them if appropriate. It means that he comes into a direct personal encounter with his client, meeting him on a person-to-person basis. It means that he is being himself, not denying himself."[49*]

This creates the opportunity for what he called "self-actualization." Carl Rogers (1959) believed that humans have one basic motive, that is the tendency to self-actualize — i.e. to fulfill one's potential and achieve the highest level of 'human-beingness' we can. "Like a flower that will grow to its full potential if the conditions are right, but which is constrained by its environment, so people will flourish and reach their potential if their environment is good enough."[50*]

Rogers has said, "constructive personality change comes about only when the client perceives and experiences a certain psychological climate in the relationship. These conditions do not consist of knowledge, intellectual training, intellectual orientation in psychotherapy, or techniques. They are feelings or attitudes which must be experienced by the therapist and perceived by the client if they are to be effective."[51]

While Rogers' focus on "congruence" was about the therapist's being congruent in themselves and with his client, I believe that the goal of any chaplaincy involvement must be to help the patient be congruent in themselves also. What Rogers spoke about as "self-actualization" is in more func-

---

49. Rogers, C. (1962 January 19). *The therapeutic relationship: Recent theory and research (p3)*. Beverly Hills, California: Los Angeles Society of Clinical Psychologists.
50. McLoed, S. (2014), Carl Rogers. Retrieved from http://www.simplypsychology.org/carl-rogers.html
*Direct quote edited for punctuation and grammar.
51. Rogers, C. (1962 January 19). *The therapeutic relationship: Recent theory and research (p6)*. Beverly Hills, California: Los Angeles Society of Clinical Psychologists.

tional and goal-oriented terms, a person becoming more congruent in themselves so that their perceived truths do not contradict each other and they do not have incongruent emotions tied to them.

When this kind of emotional and intellectual compatibility grows, it provides the opportunity for them to face the crisis with a growing peaceful acceptance, even when confronted with the prospect of death.

Basically, incongruence is tied to confusion, fear, anger, or uncertainty, which produces an unwillingness to face the future, and congruence or compatibility (self-actualization) is tied to clarity of thought and feeling, confidence, peace, and certainty with acceptance about the future.

Chaplains are focused on creating this congruence of thought and emotion, which results in better choices, greater patient satisfaction, and an easier acceptance of the reality of the situation.

Two of Fritz Perls's "Gestalt therapy" Concepts

Focus on self-awareness in the present moment by the chaplain and patient.

"According to this theory, one of the primary objectives of Gestalt therapy is the ability to restore the self-awareness which is lost when a psychological disorder becomes evident. This is accomplished by restoring the individual's ability to differentiate, which helps the individual to identify what is and what is not a true part of the self, what provides the individual with a sense of self-realization and achievement and what leads to frustration . . . His focus was to assist people in owning their experiences and developing a healthy gestalt or wholeness."[52] This was done by focusing on the present rather than on the past as Freud and Rogers did.

52. Awaken Past Teachers. (2013 January). Fritz perls. Retrieved from http://www.awaken.com/2013/01/fritz-perls/

Chaplaincy has taken this focus on the present as a key concept when connecting with others. To be truly present in that moment with the other person is a basic theme of how chaplains create a helping relationship.

Living in relationship with others is key to fully becoming the best version of yourself that you can be.

> "All people are social and they are not able to reach fully their potential without building a relationship with others and collaborating to reach the common aim. People try hard to find the harmony, peace of mind and happiness, which is unattainable on one's own, otherwise the happiness is not real. Separation from others cannot bring to genuine happiness. Happiness can be obtained in the fulfillment of real love, which is not concentrated on self but is revealed through other people to share this love with."[53]

Chaplaincy's focus on connecting with and building helpful relationships by being with another fully, in the present moment, is directly reflective of Gestalt theory.

Albert Ellis' Rational Emotive Behavior Therapy (REBT)

A person's beliefs are the key factor in facing life.

"REBT . . . is based on the premise that whenever we become upset, it is not the events taking place in our lives that upset us; it is the beliefs that we hold that cause us to become depressed, anxious, enraged, etc. The idea that our beliefs upset us was first articulated by Epictetus around 2,000 years ago: '*Men are disturbed not by events, but by the views which they take of them.*' . . . Albert Ellis and REBT posit that our reaction to having our goals blocked (or even the possibility of having them blocked) is determined by our beliefs."[54]

53. (2016). Fritz Perls. Retrieved from http://gestalttheory.com/persons/fritzperls/
54. (2006). What is REBT?. Retrieved from http://www.rebtnetwork.org/whatis.html

A persons beliefs (which they will see as an absolute truth) and the emotion that has merged with that perception are the key elements with which chaplains work when managing a patient's recovery process.

While REBT seems much like what I am talking about in this book, Ellis has emotions being only the outcome of belief and not a part of belief. REBT avoids the necessity of learning how to approach people whose first reaction to crisis is emotional rather than mental. Ellis' theory places all the work of therapists on changing beliefs by disputing the rationality of said beliefs.[55] This theory fails to explain emotions that are incongruent with a perceived truth. In other words, REBT says, beliefs, as perceived truths, result in emotions, while I am saying beliefs are perceived truths merged with emotion, resulting in convictions upon which we act. Therefore, REBT is a less effective source of care for chaplains to draw expertise from than for therapists. Ellis's theory disputes a client's irrational beliefs, whereas a chaplain's goal is not to dispute them but to gently help the patient identify the incongruences in their beliefs and make choices based on a deeper-held belief for greater congruence.

Chaplains work with a patient and/or family's beliefs as they stand in order to help them become more congruent producing better choices and greater acceptance of their situation and medical care's abilities and limitations.

Transpersonal psychology

"Relationships in transpersonal psychology are key . . . 'It is less about a particular tool or methodology and more about an intention that motivates the intervention.'"[56]

55. (2006). What is REBT?. Retrieved from http://www.rebtnetwork.org/whatis.html
56. Tartakovsky, M. (2011 November 3). 6 facts about transpersonal psychology [Blog post]. Retrieved from https://psychcentral.com/blog/archives/2011/11/03/6-facts-about-transpersonal-psychology/

Chaplains have learned that an intervention in the life and recovery of a patient and their family always requires one key ingredient to ensure success: interpersonal relationships.

A relationship is a believed mutual connection with another. A person must perceive that the other person cares about them before a relationship can be established. The same is true of a relationship between a patient and chaplain. A patient must believe that the chaplain truly cares for their well-being before they will fully connect with the chaplain. This connection must be a perceived, logical truth that has merged with an emotional feeling of closeness.

A relationship can grow quickly, like that which can form between two people who discover they are both fans of the same football team, or slowly as when points of common connection do not present themselves during initial interactions but through long-term shared experiences.

Furthermore, this connection is always in flux and is ever-changing.

Ultimately, we can say that the stresses of life can be best managed when one is in relation to another person. Feeling alone in a crisis is the greatest enemy to health.

To quote Frank Lake, "mental pain is essentially separation-anxiety, genuine relationship ends it."[57]

While much more could be said about transpersonal psychology, it is not my goal to define each stream of psychological thought but to identify key elements that are relevant to and help to further develop a chaplain's expertise. These examples of various styles of psychological thought help to illustrate the development of key concepts and language used within chaplaincy in conjunction with psychology and mental health.

---

57. Lake, F (1973) *Clinical Theology – A Theological and Psychiatric Basis to Clinical Pastoral Care* (p. 9) London, England: Darton Longman &Todd.

By examining chaplains' borrowed use of talk therapy, the therapeutic relationship, unconditional positive regard, empathy, congruence, self-actualization, self-awareness, use of self, belief, and the transformative quality of relationships, I've been lead to define spiritual care in the following manner.

Spiritual care in a medical setting is the act of

1. Building relationships with people (whether patients, families, staff, administrators or outside of hospital resources),
2. Through unconditional positive regard, empathy, and congruence
3. To help them make good choices and find comfort in those choices based on their own deepest-held beliefs
4. Because a person makes the best choices out of a conscious understanding of their own beliefs.

Chapter 8

The Belief Process of Chaplaincy vs. Evangelical Christianity

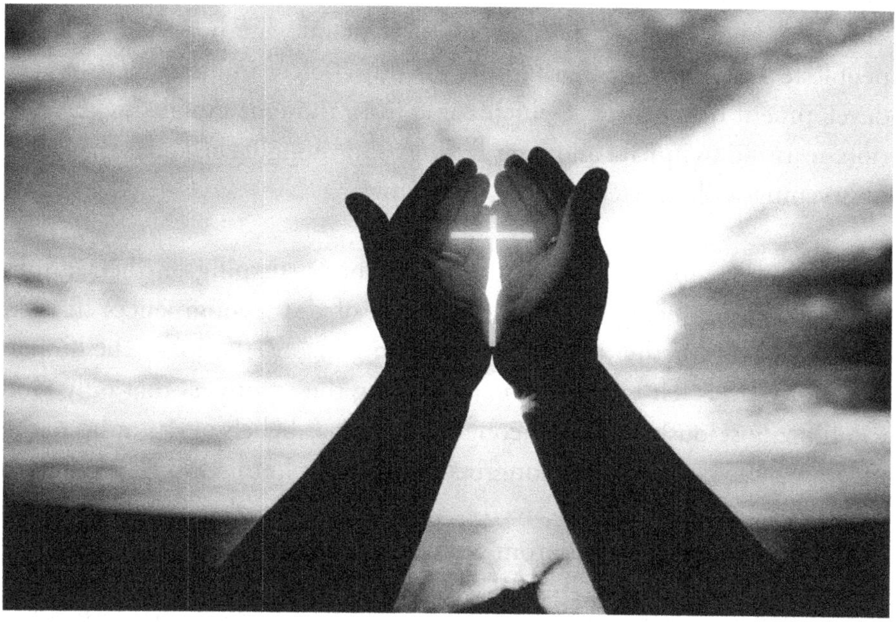

One of the questions I get most often as a chaplain is, "How can I live out my calling, as a minister, to evangelize the world (Matthew 28:19-20) when I am not allowed to proselytize in a medical setting?"

This question caused me to dig deeper into my own beliefs. I found that four beliefs were more foundational than any others in guiding my spiritual conclusions. These ideas have made me strongly evangelical in my faith while still very liberal in my approach to people, just like the Apostle Paul sought to be "all things to all people that by all means (he) might win some"(I Corinthians 9:22b).

First of all, it is important to know that evangelism is to approach people with the good news of Jesus Christ in ways that create questions about their need for Christ. According to Peter in the Bible, a Christian's job is to "always [be] prepared to make a defense to anyone who asks you for a reason for the hope that is in you; yet [to] do it with gentleness and respect"(I Peter 3:15).

The Christian Church tends to focus on the job of teaching others the Gospel and how to show the love of God to people, but not on how to help people feel the *need* for that Gospel. As our choices in life come from the development of our beliefs which come from thought mingled with emotion, learning to impact another's feelings and thoughts becomes the key to intervening without stepping on autonomy.

Remember, we impact another's beliefs without stepping on their autonomy by helping people become conscious of the incongruences in their various beliefs whether they be in their thoughts or emotions. The human need for God is felt when feeling and seeing the emptiness that only God can fill. Consciously finding incongruence in our beliefs opens us up to the only one who is completely congruent and can help us: God. The inherent quality of God lies in His perfectly congruent nature that exists even if we do not see or understand it from our incongruent, limited perspective.

Having been created in the image of God (Genesis 1:27), we have the need to be congruent in ourselves as God is. This need for congruency is what many Christians speak about as the hole that only God can fill in their life.

This need for congruence has been identified in psychology as "a consistent state of behavior, meaning there is consistency between the goals, values, and attitudes projected and the actual behavior observed. In personality research, ideally, the way you think and feel should also be the way you behave."[58]

I would argue that this need is not just for a consistency between ones "goals, values, and attitudes projected and the actual behavior observed," but also the need for ones goals, values and attitudes being consistent to one's feelings and to each other. The need for congruence in every aspect of one's life comes from being created in the image of a totally congruent God.

Secondly, many Christians think that evangelism is just a matter of finding better ways of explaining who Jesus is and what He comes to do. Yet, without a person feeling the need for God, they do not have much of an interest in God and are not therefore drawn to God anyways. In other words, if I do not consciously see and feel my own incongruences, I will neither see nor feel the need for the congruent God who is seeking to have a relationship with me and satisfy my needs. Without the benefit of experiencing an open, honest, congruent relationship with another person, it becomes impossible to believe in a true relationship with God who is totally congruent. Being ready to explain the reason for the hope that we have is predicated on a question being asked. Those questions come from touching another's life with congruence.

Thirdly, God is seeking us (Luke 19:10, Revelation 3:20) and only He can lead us to the conviction of our need for Christ (John 16:8-11). No great argument will convince if one does not see and feel the need for themselves first, for choices are made out of our beliefs that are perceived truths tied to emotions.

Finally, the groundwork for seeing one's need for change can be found in the conscious recognition that what one believes about something is incongruent or ineffective. As I seek to make it congruent, I will find that, apart from God I cannot find the congruency I seek (John 15:5). I will therefore

58. Nugent, P. (2013 April 7). Behavioral congruence. Retrieved from http://psychology-dictionary.org/behavioral-congruence

ultimately be drawn to God in my honest search for what is good (Proverbs 11:27), for everything good comes from God (James 1:17).

As a chaplain I may not have the same duty of proclaiming the good news of Jesus Christ as pastors do, but I do have the same responsibility that pastors have to help people see their need for something greater than themselves (which is a spiritual/belief activity) by recognizing the incongruences in their lives.

This incongruence in itself calls to people and tells them that something more is needed.

While psychotherapeutic thought has identified many truths about how one can intervene in another's life without stepping on their autonomy (See Chapter 7), these same truths have been present in the Bible since before people recognized them and tried to define them separately from the Bible.

The following is a review of some of the parallels between what the Bible has said for centuries and modern psychological thought as presented in Chapter 7.

When Freud promoted the idea of "talk therapy," he was only thinking on a human level, but wasn't aware of how God always approaches us as "the Word" (John 1:1) and is seeking to have a conversational relationship with us (Genesis 3:8-24 & John 1:1).

When Carl Rogers promoted his psychotherapy interventions, they were always based on his three secularized concepts of "Unconditional Positive Regard," "Empathy," and "Congruence" (see Chapter 7). These he developed after leaving seminary, rejecting religious thought and becoming a humanist.[59] Yet, these concepts are clearly paralleled by the Love of God (1John 4:7-12, Romans 5:7-10) and His unconditional positive regard for

59. Esbensen, J. Carl Rogers. Retrieved from https://ffrf.org/news/day/famous-freethinkers-secular-stars/spotlight/item/14134-carl-rogers

us by wanting all to be saved (2 Peter 3:9), by Christ coming to Earth to be "tempted in all ways, yet without sin" thereby being able to empathize with us as humans (Hebrews 4:15), and by the immutability of God's holiness proving His true congruence in all matters — "The outer expression and the inward reality always correspond"[60].

The Christian church has often done a good job of training its members on how to proclaim the good news about Jesus Christ, but has often failed to help people really perceive and feel the need for Christ.

People's incongruence, when recognized, draws them to seek congruence from the very God in whose image we were created.

The world's answers fall short of creating true congruence. God is ready to have a relationship with us and teach us true congruence, as He is the only being that is truly congruent and therefore the only one able to teach it without error.

Helping people find God starts with helping them to recognize their incongruence and having a congruent relationship with them. This creates the question of the proposed source of a potential greater congruence. We then, when asked, have an obligation to explore the question together.

60. Strong, A. (1972), *Systematic theology* (P. 288). Valley Forge, PA: Judson Press.

[illegible]

[illegible]

[illegible]

[illegible]

[illegible]

[illegible]

Chapter 9

How to Approach Beliefs Without Stepping on Autonomy

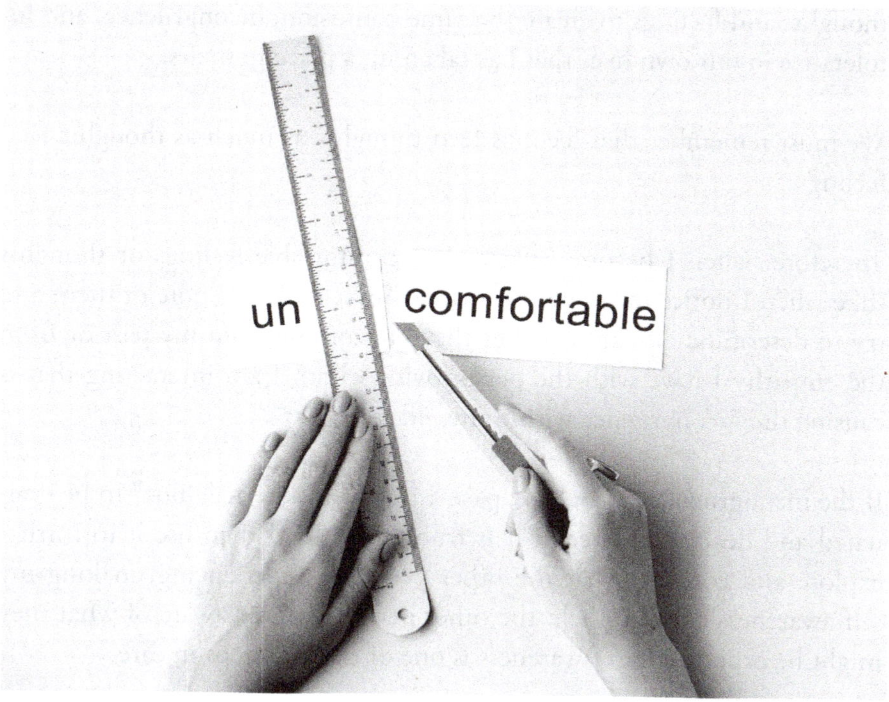

Become Comfortable With Being Uncomfortable

When we become uncomfortable because we encounter a type of situation or a type of person we have not yet had experience with or do not like, we tend to cut short or leave the encounter or want to try to coerce them into believing as we do. In order to become comfortable with being uncomfortable, we must identify our own sources of discomfort and push ourselves to remain in a situation and understand the other party's discomfort as well.

This will grow an assurance that we have the ability to face anything life can throw at us without it dragging us down. A chaplain's expertise is the ability to empathize with another's feelings without having the same fear, anger, or loneliness empathically invade our souls. As chaplains, we must be able to understand another person's feelings, seeking to know them as God does, without having those same feelings become a part of our lives, out of empathy. We must be able to be completely emotionally, mentally, and physically present, without allowing the impact of the other person's thoughts and feelings to create the same confusion, incongruence, and intolerance in our own lives that has taken up a place in theirs.

We must remember that feelings feed thoughts as much as thoughts feed feelings.

Therefore, when I become aware of uncomfortable feelings or thoughts (like when I notice incongruence within myself), I take note of them and try to determine quickly whether they are coming from my past or from the empathy I have with the person with whom I am interacting that is causing the incongruence within myself.

If the incongruence is from my past, I put in an internal "box" to be evaluated and dealt with later. If it is from empathy, I then use it to further explore and confirm what the other person is experiencing, making my self-awareness a tool to help the other person become aware of what they might be experiencing. Awareness is one of the first steps in care.

Be cautious about using questions

Doctors and psychiatrists have such limited time availability that they must try to get at the crux of the issues as quickly as possible by asking questions in order to diagnose the problem.

Chaplains, however, are not so much diagnosticians as facilitators of self-discovery and encouragers of autonomy. We help people become aware of their own beliefs and make choices based on those beliefs in a world that has taught them to try to manipulate each other's choices for their own benefit.

Questions are often used to manipulate others in our society. Therefore, people usually put up their guard when asked a question, making it harder to connect with them beyond the cursory niceties.

When you ask a question, you are directing the other person to think in the direction of the question rather than inviting them to freely share what is going on within their life, mind, and emotions.

This is why I work to simply understand and verbally reflect what I see in front of me; instead of asking questions and skewing the answers with the way the questions are phrased; I practice reflective listening.

Most questions are formed based on something we think might be happening without checking to be sure with the patient. While questions can be used to check the accuracy of what we perceive, reflecting without asking questions is a less directive approach.

If we back up one step and check what we hear or see by reflecting what we recognize in them, we become less directive and give the patient the opportunity to affirm or reject our perceptions without embarrassment. By asking questions, the other person is not only put on their guard but becomes fearful of not answering in the right way. With reflection, the other person is given the power to accept or reject the tentative perception, and I am the one who has the possibility of being wrong rather than the patient.

"How are you feeling today?" becomes, "You look tired, worn out, or alert, etc., today." If they are feeling contrarily, they are more likely to correct you rather than feel affronted or made afraid by a question.

Questions can potentially be helpful when exploring an issue already identified and affirmed by a patient, but they need to be used sparingly or as a vehicle for strengthening a person's sense of autonomy. A question like "How do you face such an issue?" gives the control of the choices and situation back to the patient. "How can you do such a thing?" takes the control away from the patient as the question manipulates the other's feelings and responses through judgmental tone.

Because we are taught in our society how to subconsciously manipulate each other with the way we pose our questions, it is much harder to use questions in an open, honest way, than to use reflective listening that does not say, "Are you saying…?" but rather, "I hear you saying…"

Loss of control and the sense of being alone are two of the biggest enemies in healthcare for patients, families and friends, and staff. Manipulation seeks to take control and autonomy away from the patient which further advances the feelings of being alone.

Seek the emotions of the situation

We often think in terms of what may or may not be true, and therefore have become skilled in thinking in terms of intervention. However, we generally have much less skill in being with a person on an emotional level because it makes us uncomfortable. This can be most easily seen in the urge to speak in the middle of a long silence. We want to fill the void with words and thoughts rather than sit and just be with another emotionally.

To reflect what another might be experiencing emotionally can be done with words, but is often better fulfilled with a touch, silence, a look, a deep breath, company, and so on.

It is on an emotional level where we can always connect with another, even when we personally, deeply disagree with their choices, beliefs, or actions.

I remember once sitting with a homosexual person who had woken up that morning and found their partner dead in the bed beside them. 911 responded and brought the person and their partner to the emergency room, doing CPR for a time, until finally pronouncing the partner dead. As I sat with them in the family room, knowing from the medical team that there had been no signs of life, I knew I could not congruently connect with the partner on their lifestyle choices but I could with how it would feel to wake up and find my wife dead in the bed next to me. These feelings became the basis upon which I prepared him for the news the doctors would probably bring shortly. He shared how their families had abandoned them because of their choices and how difficult it was going to be to contact the partner's family about what had happened. I did not have to bring up any questions as the conversation naturally flowed out of his expression of feelings. The feelings of fear and pain at the loss of his partner were interwoven with the fear and pain at the loss of family. This helped him become able to contact family, even though neither wanted to see the other, and I was able to provide help to the mother, who came in later. I empathically connected with them both on an emotional level without erecting a barrier within me that might keep me from connecting with either him or the mother.

The crisis of the present moment requires congruent emotional connection and after that, congruence of thinking will be needed as choices are made.

Congruence, or lack thereof, in approaching people will always be emotionally sensed by others

One of the things that has struck me the most about caring for people in medical situations is that they can always sense whether I am fully present and caring about them as human beings. Using Rogers' and/or a Biblical concept, one could say people can always sense whether you have "unconditional positive regard", i.e. the love of God, for them or not. Whether you are truly present with them or are distracted by something (like the list of people you still have to see) will always be felt even if unrecognized.

The wariness of being easily hurt in a crisis and our walls being stripped down by that crisis creates an unconscious sensitivity to whether we as chaplains are truly there for the other or just doing a job.

One final glimpse at the effects of a chaplain's expertise

It was early in my chaplain residency. She was in her 40s with a very active mind but had not spoken for three years following a brain injury.

I decided to visit her for a length of time after hearing from a nurse about her situation and reflecting on the implications of not being able to speak for so long.

I spoke to her about how I sensed that people don't visit for very long but just come in and do their job because they don't know how to relate to a person who is so active mentally but cannot speak.

Her face, very expressively, affirmed that people always seemed in a hurry to get out of the room. This even extended to the way her family related to her unfortunately.

I offered her my hand, which she took and held strongly, as I told her that I wanted to spend time with her since others were not. For 20 minutes I reflected to her how I imagine it must be to not be able to speak when one has so much to say. She affirmed much of what I was sensing with her face and gestures and shook her head when what I said was not true to her experience.

Even when reflecting on my holding her hand for a longer time than anyone had done for some time, she winked at me and nodded strongly while squeezing my hand in appreciation.

At times, I spoke of what I was sensing while she reflected back with facial expressions, and at others, we just sat looking into each other's eyes while holding hands. We were connected, even when in silence, without embarrassment or questioning.

At the end of those 20 minutes I gave my good-bye and as I left she said, "Thank you."

These were the first words she had spoken in three years.

It was then I learned the impact that chaplaincy can have on another's life beyond medicine if we but congruently seek to connect with others with a willingness to sit with them in their world that is often much different than our own.

Chapter 10

Conclusion

We are motivated to make the choices we make when our thoughts and feelings merge into convictions. Neither thoughts nor feelings carry greater weight when developing our convictions upon which we make choices in life. Convictions develop at the point that the two merge together to form a belief.

At this merging point is where, we as chaplains, must stand ready to connect either first through thoughts or feelings in order to help a person in crisis explore the fullness of their beliefs and help make more congruent those beliefs, for better choices. Choices demanded by the crisis of the present or future medical crisis.

It is the autonomy of the other person that we are always fighting for as we interact in order to build the other persons resiliency, through congruent beliefs, so that they are able to not only make choices consistent with their deepest held beliefs but also stand against those who wish to impose their desires on them in opposition to their own beliefs.

I have grown, through chaplaincy, to realize that it is the emotional part of belief that connects or disconnects people to each other more than thought. Yet, in our society we are poorly taught how to interact emotionally and often find it hard to spend much time reflecting on our emotions. I still find it easier to reflect on what I *think* about the world around me and God than on how I personally *feel* about it all.

Yet, as I have grown in my abilities to recognize and reflect back my own and others emotions, I have found that I can more easily share those emotions of a good cry or laugh.

Chaplaincy for me has been the pinnacle of ministry. It has helped me to more clearly understand God's plan for me in life. My life's feeling of completeness has grown as I have looked back and discovered that, as God was using me in peoples' medical crises, so He had been using me in the crises of the churches at which I had served as a pastor, of the units for which I served as an Air Force Chaplain, and the situations into which I found myself as a police chaplain. By reviving the churches threatened by demise or exponential growth, preparing airmen for the trauma of war, and helping police and the public face the unexpected events that threatened to crush them, I, too, was being helped.

I found myself to be at my most helpful when I simply sat with a wife as her husband was in surgery, when I asked a family about their loved one whose funeral I was preparing and listened to their stories, when I cried with those in tears, when I answered their questions rather than asking my own, when I gave over control to another person, or when I stopped trying to fix others and let God do the fixing.

My chaplaincy journey has been one of self-discovery in a world that tries to make us too busy for that discovery; a discovery in which one does not need to have the answers in order to be of help to another, but just needs to be willing to be with a person when they are facing the trauma and crisis that life brings.

Bibliography

(2006). What is REBT? Retrieved from http://www.rebtnetwork.org/whatis.html

About Spiritual Care Association (2017). Retrieved from https://www.spiritualcareassociation.org

Awaken Past Teachers. (2013, January). Fritz Perls. Retrieved from http://www.awaken.com/2013/01/fritz-perls/

Awaken Past Teachers. (2016). Fritz Perls. Retrieved from http://gestalttheory.com/persons/fritzperls/

Benight, C., Swift, E., Sanhger, J., Smith, A., & Zeppelin, D. (1999). Coping self-efficacy as a mediator of distress following a natural disaster. Journal of Applied Social Psychology, 29, 2443-2464.

Boisen, A. T. (2005). The Living Human Document. In Robert C. Dykstra (Ed.), *Images of Pastoral Care, Classic Readings* (p.22-29). St. Louis, Missouri: Chalice Press.

Bradberry, T. & Greaves, J. (2015). Emotional intelligence 2.0. Retrieved from http://www.talentsmart.com/products/emotional-intelligence-2.0/

Bradberry, T. (2015, January 7). Why you need emotional intelligence. Retrieved from https://www.forbes.com/sites/travisbradberry/2015/01/07/why-you-need-emotional-intelligence-to-succeed/#7574ffda6246/

Campbell, A. V. (2005). The Courageous Shepherd. In Robert C. Dykstra (Ed.), *Images of Pastoral Care, Classic Readings* (p.54-61). St. Louis, Missouri: Chalice Press.

Capps, D. (2005). The Agent of Hope. In Robert C. Dykstra (Ed.), *Images of Pastoral Care, Classic Readings* (p.188-199). St. Louis, Missouri: Chalice Press.

Dollars in detail. Retrieved from https://www.uscurrency.gov/sites/default/files/download-materials/en/CEP_Dollars_In_Detail_Brochure.pdf

Dykstra, R. C. (2005). The Intimate Stranger. In Robert C. Dykstra (Ed.), *Images of Pastoral Care, Classic Readings* (p.123-136). St. Louis, Missouri: Chalice Press.

Epstien, R. M. & Street, R. L. Jr. (2011). The Values and Value of Patient-Centered Care. *Annals of Family Medicine*, 9/2, (p.100-103).

Esbensen, J. Carl Rogers. Retrieved from https://ffrf.org/news/day/famous-freethinkers-secular-stars/spotlight/item/14134-carl-rogers

Everly, G.S. Jr & Mitchell, J.T. (1997*). Critical incident stress management - A new era and standard of care in crisis intervention.* Ellicott City, MD: Chevron Publishing Corporation.

Everly, G.S. Jr. & Mitchell, J.F. (2008). *Integrative crisis intervention and disaster mental health.* Ellicott City, MD: Chevron Publishing Corporation.

Faber, H (2005). The Circus Clown. In Robert C. Dykstra (Ed.), *Images of Pastoral Care, Classic Readings* (p.85-93). St. Louis, Missouri: Chalice Press.

Frampton, S., Guastello S., Brady, C., Hale, M., Horowitz, S. Smith, S.B. & Stone S. (2008 October). *Patient-centered care improvement guide (*p.3)

Fromme, E.K. & Arnold, R.M. (2011), Approaching patients and family members who hope for a miracle, *Journal of Pain and Symptom Management,* Abstract. Retrieved from http://www.jpsmjournal.com/article/S0885-3924(11)00243-0/fulltext

Gadjanski, K, The importance of a therapeutic relationship - in psychotherapy and beyond. Retrieved from www.chiswickhomeopathyclinic.co.uk/TherapeuticRelationship. Artic..doc

Hall, E.J., Hughes B.P., Handzo, G.H. (2016, October). *Spiritual care: what it means, why it matters in health care. Retrieved from* https://www.healthcarechaplaincy.org/docs/about/spirituality.pdf

Healthcare Chaplaincy Network. Retrieved from https://healthcarechaplaincy.org/clinical-pastoral-education.html

History of psychotherapy. Retrieved from https://en.wikipedia.org/wiki/History_of_psychotherapy

How does the FBI train agents to spot counterfeit money? Retrieved from http://www.answers.com/Q/How_does_the_FBI_train_agents_to_spot_counterfeit_money?#slide=2

Lake, F (1973) *Clinical Theology – A Theological and Psychiatric Basis to Clinical Pastoral Care* (p. 9) London, England: Darton Longman &Todd.

Langstrom, M. W. & Langstrom, K. J. (2016). *A journey to hope – healing the traumatized spirit.* Silverton, OR: Lampion Press.

Lichter, D.A. & O'Gorman, M.L. (2009, May-June). Establishing a chaplain's value. Retrieved from https://www.chausa.org/pastoralcare/resources/pastoral-care-articles/may-june-2009/establishing-a-chaplain's-value

Lipka, M. (2015, May 13), A closer look at America's rapidly growing religious 'nones'. Retrieved from http://pewresearch.org/fact-tank/2015/05/13/a-closer-look-at-american-rapidely-growing-religious-nones

McLoed, S. (2014), Carl Rogers. Retrieved from http://www.simplypsychology.org/carl-rogers.html

Myers, D., & Wee, D.F. (2005). *Disaster mental Health services* (p.12, 26) New York, NY: Routledge Taylor & Francis Group.

Nouwen, H. J. M. (2005). The Wounded Healer. In Robert C. Dykstra (Ed.), *Images of Pastoral Care, Classic Readings* (p.76-84). St. Louis, Missouri: Chalice Press.

Nugent, P. (2013, April 7). Behavioral congruence. Retrieved from http://psychologydictionary.org/behavioral-congruence

Pew Research Center. (2012, October 9). Retrieved from http://www.pewforum.org/2012/10/09/nones-on-the-rise

Pew Research Center. (2015, May 12). America's changing religious landscape. Retrieved from http://www.pewforum.org/2015/05/12/americas-changing-religious-landscape/

Pruyser, P. W. (2005). The Diagnostician. In Robert C. Dykstra (Ed.), *Images of Pastoral Care, Classic Readings* (pp.161-170). St. Louis, Missouri: Chalice Press.

Rice, S. (2015). Most hospitals face 30-day readmissions penalty in fiscal 2016. *Modern healthcare* http://www.modernhealthcare.com/article/20150803/NEWS/150809981/

Roberts, S. B. (2012). Professional Spiritual & Pastoral Care (p.24). Skylight Paths Publishing, Woodstock, Vermont: Skylight Paths Publishing.

Rogers, C. (1962, January 19). *The therapeutic relationship: Recent theory and research* (p.3-6). Beverly Hills, California: Los Angeles Society of Clinical Psychologists.

Simons, S.G. (2008, January 1), Grace notes. Retrieved from http://www.e-gracenotes.org/article/2673/archives/the-bible-says/the-real-thing

Skanse, J. E. (2009). The power of touch. *Plainviews*, 6/18. http://www.plainviews.org

Skanse, J. E. (2010). Finding a Reason To Be. *Plainviews*, 7/18. http://www.plainviews.org

Strong, A. (1972), *Systematic theology* (p.288). Valley Forge, PA: Judson Press.

Tartakovsky, M. (2011, November 3). 6 facts about Transpersonal Psychology [Blog post]. Retrieved from: https://psychcentral.com/blog/archives/2011/11/03/6-facts-about-transpersonal-psychology/

US Department of Veterans Affairs, PTSD: National Center for PTSD. How common is PTSD? Retrieved from https://www.ptsd.va.gov/public/PTSD-overview/basics/how-common-is-ptsd.asp

US Department of Veterans Affairs, PTSD: National Center for PTSD. Common reactions after trauma. Retrieved from https://www.ptsd.va.gov/public/problems/common-reactions-after-trauma.asp

Wieman, R. (2015, July 7). Sigmund Freud (1856-1939). Retrieved from http://www.goodtherapy.org/famous-psychologists/sigmund-freud.html

Acknowledgments

I wish to thank Chaplain Andy Leatherman who encouraged me to delve further into a person's emotions beyond their thoughts. I'd also like to thank all the chaplain interns at Einstein who encouraged me over the years to write this book based on the classes I taught on the subject.

Acknowledgments

[illegible] K. Chaplin, Andy Cushman, who [illegible] professors [illegible] beyond [illegible] [illegible] through [illegible] [illegible] of this book based on [illegible]

Index

About the Author

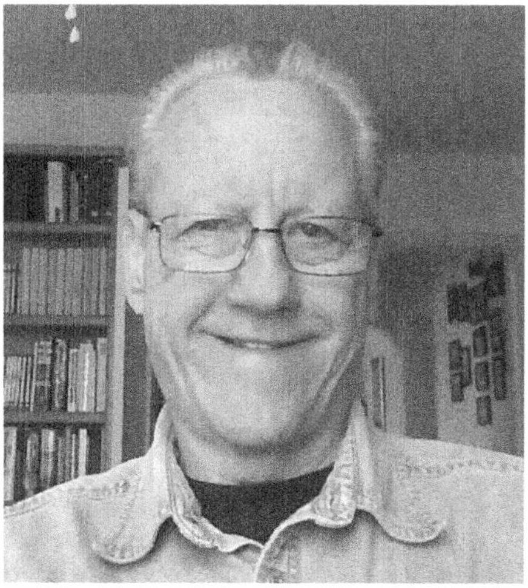

Chaplain John E. Skanse has a B.A. in Christian Education, a certificate from the Evangelical Teacher Training Association, and an M.Div in Pastoral Care with a focus on counseling, in addition to many other certifications and qualifications. After 30 years of pastoring, 20 of which he also spent as an Air Force Chaplain with the Illinois Air National Guard, he went on to spend four and half years as a Police Chaplain. He then became a Trauma/Emergency Staff Chaplain at Einstein Medical Center (EMC) and then chaplaincy palliative care coordinator.

Chaplain Skanse retired in 2016 and began writing this work in an attempt to further flesh out concepts on chaplaincy he had first published in PlainViews.

Made in the USA
Monee, IL
04 November 2026

67386399R10056